# Psychic

## How to Develop Your Inner Psychic Power

*(Shield Yourself From Toxic Energy and Prevent Psychic Attacks)*

### Charles Centers

Published By **Andrew Zen**

## Charles Centers

*Psychic: How to Develop Your Inner Psychic Power
(Shield Yourself From Toxic Energy and Prevent
Psychic Attacks)*

**ISBN   978-1-998927-99-9**

No part of this guidebook shall be reproduced in any form without permission in writing from the publisher except in the case of brief quotations embodied in critical articles or reviews.

Legal & Disclaimer

The information contained in this book is not designed to replace or take the place of any form of medicine or professional medical advice. The information in this book has been provided for educational & entertainment purposes only.

The information contained in this book has been compiled from sources deemed reliable, and it is accurate to the best of the Author's knowledge; however, the Author cannot guarantee its accuracy and validity and cannot be held liable for any errors or omissions. Changes are periodically made to this book. You must consult your doctor or get professional medical advice before using any of the suggested remedies, techniques, or information in this book.

Table Of Contents

# Chapter 1: The History Of Psychics

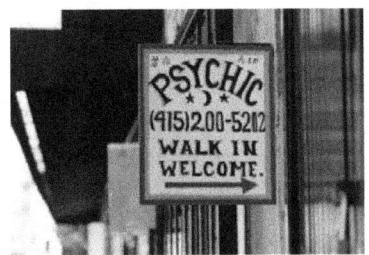

Some of the primary evidence of psychics dates again to the Roman Empire. At the time, they have been known as clairvoyants and labored as advisors. It is said that the psychics had an instantaneous connection to the gods and goddesses. They could speak to them and tell the kings and queens about their messages. Psychics have been a large part of the selection-making method. They had been consulted for each choice, irrespective of how massive or small. This blanketed the decision to go to conflict, to gain and plant vegetation, and take authorities action. Sadly, this additionally got here at a value. If the selection that changed into made based at the psychic's opinion failed, the psychic may want to frequently be jailed or sentenced to dying.

A psychic's position stepped forward as civilization stepped forward. When tribes commenced out to form, shamans possessed psychic abilities. They have emerge as the number one medical medical doctors of villages. Once over again, shamans carried out a completely essential function inside the society. They have been usually present at ceremonies to offer cosmic energy. They should perform divination—the practice of seeing the destiny or answering questions—the usage of clairvoyance or out-of-frame evaluations.

Eventually, psychics started out to use gadgets to sell the conjuring of spiritual strength. When a psychic had advanced their powers, they'll begin to use equipment collectively with jewels, crystals, bones, and divining rods. They have to use them to encourage greater power. Dice and dominoes in the interim are typical as powerful gear for advanced psychic readings.

Psychics moreover evolved the idea of fulfillment. They defined that there isn't proper achievement or awful excellent fortune; it is all honestly energy. The power round you controls the final results in some situations. Most human beings aren't aware of the form of strength they will be liberating into the universe. This energy ultimately finally ends up reflecting once more on them, each truely or negatively. This is an critical reason why you ought to discover ways to understand and manipulate your competencies.

With the upward push of prepared religious society, the popularity of psychic capacity disappeared. Jewish, Christian, and Islamic leaders all proclaimed that psychics were not anything extra than witches or evil beings. Religious leaders began out to worry that the potential to expect may motive them to lose control of their congregations. Foretelling, similar to psychic instinct, is the capability to experience what is going to take vicinity. Religious leaders feared they may now not be visible because the people with connections to higher beings. This introduced approximately psychics being banished, sent to jail, or killed.

One of the most well-known historic recollections of psychics is the Salem Witch Trials. From February 1692 to May 1693, a collection of women happy a whole village that quite a few its citizens were witches. It started out with Betty Parris, nine, and Abigail Williams, 11, experiencing "suits" that they blamed on witchcraft. Women and men had been sentenced to lack of life for their meant paintings with the devil. In all, 19 human beings have been hanged, plenty of them women. One seventy one-365 days-antique guy became pressed to demise, and numerous humans died in jail, of whom had been infants. Nearly hundred human beings were accused of being witches. The Christian church helped lead the Salem Witch Trials because it felt that psychic ability changed into an insult to their creator. Luckily, a trendy courtroom docket end up positioned into place and nearly definitely anyone had their expenses absolved and were given yet again their actual names.

Fortunately, now psychics are an ordinary a part of society. That's no longer to say there aren't those who despite the fact that don't consider on this shape of issue. Police departments are actually employing psychics to assist them treatment crimes.

Scientific research has demonstrated that psychic skills are real, and are now a place of test. Research has proven that psychic talents are just like the energy determined in quantum physics. Psychics have even made it onto TV suggests as vital characters, and it's hard not to discover a ebook on the trouble.

Religious leaders despite the fact that disapprove of psychic skills. They even though warn their flocks about the evil doings of psychics, writing them off as frauds, con artists, or satan worshipers. Despite the developing amount of evidence that such abilities do exist, psychics continue to be unwanted traffic in masses of non secular institutions.

Psychic Intuition

Intuition is the feeling of being pulled in a fine route, which commonly can't be described. Most of the time, humans consult with this as a gut intuition, just like while you meet a person new and get a revel in about whether you can like them. You also can check it as your internal voice or better self this is associated with something larger inside the universe. When you can quiet your mind, your voice becomes clearer and louder. Being psychic is having extra unique intuitive statistics. It helps construct greater from your intuition, making it clearer and imparting you with greater notion. The facts you get preserve of may be through clairvoyance, clairaudience, clairsentience, claircognizance, or clairgustance. Instead of having a gut feeling about whether you may like a person, you'll get a photo or apprehend a detail from their existence.

The first of the 4 maximum critical intuitive capabilities is clairvoyance, because of this smooth seeing. It is the most commonplace form of psychic intuition. Clairvoyance is the functionality to see something for your mind's eye. It's like seeing a film inner your head. It doesn't endorse you are seeing the future or a few aspect most crucial; it may from time to time be subtle. You might probable see handiest a shade, quite a variety of, or a photo. It can be as lots as you to figure out what they imply but they may be complete-blown premonitions.

The 2nd potential is clairsentience, because of this that easy feeling. Clairsentience manner you can gain intuitive messages by way of feelings, emotions, or sensations. Empathy is a commonplace shape of clairsentience. These varieties of humans frequently find out themselves feeling pretty tired due to the fact they will be constantly bombarded with the aid of terrible and splendid feelings and feelings. You can also stroll as tons as everybody you slightly recognize and comprehend exactly how they experience. Clairsentience additionally gives you the capability to understand if someone is lying to you, that could are available in accessible. If your competencies are very strong, you may even start to experience ill even as others near you're sick.

The 1/3 capability is clairaudience, because of this clear paying attention to. It's a way to receive messages with out the usage of your physical ear. Just like clairvoyance is inner seeing, clairaudience is inner taking note of. Maybe you have got were given heard any man or woman assist you to recognize a few thing however no person is around you, or the individual you are with didn't say some issue. Psychics will pay attention a spirit speakme to them of their heads. It will sound like even as you're analyzing silently to yourself. On some activities, they may listen the voice inside the accessory of the person speakme to them.

The fourth potential is claircognizance, which means that smooth knowledge. This is the capability to recognize a few trouble whilst no longer having statistics or records. You may additionally additionally truly recognize that you shouldn't consider your new neighbor or a person who virtually started taking walks on your workplace. These emotions can be tremendously robust and pop into your head at random times. You can also have had some of the ones thoughts earlier than. Maybe you have been on the point of get on the elevator however a belief popped into your head and informed you to take the stairs. Then you located out later that the elevator had gotten stuck.

One of the less not unusual and much less-identified psychic intuitions is clairalience, which is apparent smelling. This is the capability to odor past the ordinary flair. An example is if you're at domestic and perfume fragrance, a cigar, or any fragrance you associate with a deceased relative. Another a terrific deal less not unusual capability is clairgustance, because of this clean tasting. This is the capacity to flavor a few thing earlier than you positioned it to your mouth. It is typically experienced thru mediums all through a studying. When a psychic is making an attempt to talk with an entity, they're capable of start developing a flavor in their mouth. For example, if the entity they're seeking to acquire desired chocolate once they were alive, the psychic should possibly start to flavor chocolate.

These are a few examples of psychic instinct. You do no longer need to hold these varieties of abilities. You may additionally furthermore have handiest one or two, and you could end up having they all at numerous instances counting on how an entity wishes to speak with you.

## Chapter 2: Early Signs And Types Of Psychic Abilities

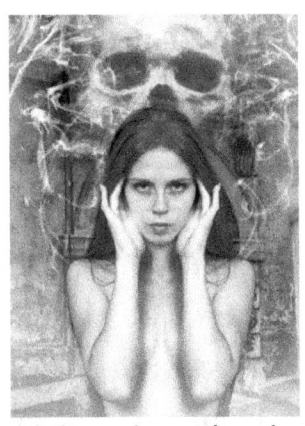

Psychic capability doesn't play favorites. It's no longer something handiest positive people could have. There is a extensive type of power in terms of someone's psychic potential. This may additionally need to suggest which you have some thing from a sense that someone goes to call you to an potential to look at different people's emotions and thoughts. Research has examined that everyone is born able to increase psychic abilities. Researchers have moreover decided that ancestry and children play a huge characteristic in whether or not the capacity develops on its very non-public or whether or not or no longer one need to growth their very non-public.

Ancestry

It's believed that one's family records performs a large characteristic in figuring out whether or now not a infant is greater vulnerable to being psychic. To add to this, during the time at the same time as villages used shamans, the shaman's infant might have a look at to take over after his father's dying. Another instance of families playing a huge component in psychic ability is sisters Kate and Maggie Fox, who worked together to determined Spiritualism. They have been each superior psychics. Spiritualism is verbal exchange with the spirits of the useless.

A have a have a look at in Scotland led through Shari Cohn started analyzing the patterns amongst families inside the Highlands and Western Isles of Scotland. She placed that the numerous households regarded to have the capabilities of second sight (that is being capable of see activities in remote places wherein the psychic is not gift), retro-cognition (seeing the beyond), and precognition (seeing the future). Two hundred and eight people had been studied and Cohn decided that a massive percent of the population possessed psychic talents. She additionally confirmed that ladies had been more likely to be psychic, and if someone had a twin, or had twins of their circle of relatives, they have been more likely to be psychic.

Additionally, Cohn's studies confirmed that families that had psychic competencies and believed in them, encouraging their use, had an prolonged line of psychics. Sylvia Wright moreover confirmed this relation. In families wherein psychic capabilities aren't believed in or supported via the family, kids generally repress their competencies, whilst kids with families that assist and encourage them could have robust psychic abilties.

One psychic spoke with a sociologist and, during their interview, told them how one night at the equal time as she have become a infant, she advised her mother that someone become popularity in the nook of her room. Her mother answered through asking, "What is his call?"

In a few different story, a psychic knowledgeable how her grandmother used to help her decorate her potential with video games, which incorporates hiding a key in her residence and telling her to "be the critical element, then see in that you're."

## Damaging Childhood

Stress and trauma professional in adolescence are one of a kind sturdy factors in developing psychic capability. A researcher who had interviewed several psychics and mediums over numerous years said that nearly every person interviewed had skilled some form of personal trauma of their childhoods. The University of Chicago determined comparable results while interviewing psychics. Its look at confirmed that youngsters who expert anxiety of their households or who had a difficult courting with a parent (the father more so than the mother) had been more likely to develop psychic ability. Interestingly, these subjects had an above-average score for his or her present day lifestyles pleasure. The quit modified into that psychic abilities had a correlation to difficult upbringings, but didn't affect happiness in person life.

Science explains this as "use it or lose it." We are born with hundreds of hundreds of mind cells. As we grow up, if these cells aren't used, they may die off. What you experience sooner or later of young people dictates what mind cells can be saved, normally earlier than the age of 10. The thoughts's business enterprise is managed with the resource of the manner the cells expand. If a child indicates psychic talents, encouraging them will inform the mind to maintain using the ones thoughts cells, permitting the child's abilities to expand. Not using them will cause the ones cells to die off.

Proteins are produced when genes are allowed to be expressed, which in flip develops genes, cells, and neurons. When a little one who has a predisposition in the path of being a psychic is supported and helped to enhance their psychic capabilities, extra pathways are created in the mind, thinking of further development. Genes that guide psychic skills are observed essentially inside the prefrontal cortex. The cortex will preserve growing in supported, clever children till across the age of 11 or 12.

Psychologists have studied the reasoning at the back of psychic ability due to trauma. They say that after youngsters are put in a worrying scenario, the thoughts commonly disassociates from its environment. For safety, it'll divert the child an extended way from aware fact. Disassociating permits the thoughts to song into specific realities, possibly even extraordinary worlds, locations, and times. In some studies, adults who had professional annoying activities as kids recalled having out-of-frame reviews. One such psychic said that physical abuse happened nearly each day. She stated that in the abuse, she wouldn't hear or enjoy a few aspect, in spite of the reality that she knew and could see what end up happening. She would turn out to be numb to get away.

Another take a look at explaining kids pressure-precipitated psychic capability looked at children of alcoholics or drug addicts. AL-ANON is a hard and fast for person kids of addicts. The agency frequently talks about the notion of others' emotions, commonly parents. One participant, at some point of a take a look at in 1999, stated that usually he may arrive domestic not information whether or not his mother grow to be surpassed out somewhere. As he walked into the house, earlier than he ever saw her, he need to tell what his mom's cutting-edge-day nation have become. He unconsciously knowledgeable himself to have a have a look at her thoughts and moods absolutely so he need to understand whilst she changed into much more likely to turn out to be irrational and risky. This is called being a psychic empath—being capable of sense the ache and emotions of others. Instead of disassociation, youngsters who boom this acquire this as a method of self-renovation.

Some precise predictors for psychic talents are if a child modified into raised by means of manner of authoritarian, strict, or abusive dad and mom, which encompass unloving dad and mom who forced and demanded total obedience. Other predictors are if a toddler out of location their mother, had an excessive contamination or deformity that required some of corrective surgical strategies or had dad and mom who every suffered from bi-polar sickness. The danger of having psychic capacity is heightened with a mixture of stressors and circle of relatives facts.

Studies show that everybody is born with the possibility to own psychic tendencies, however they normally require a cause, like younger people trauma, a stressor, or own family statistics. This generally have to reveal up earlier than age 10 for the frontal lobe to thicken, allowing synapses and neurons to shape. An exception is if the child is extraordinarily clever, owning a immoderate IQ; in this case, they've till the age of 12 for the frontal lobe adjustments to take vicinity. There are greater psychic girls who came from families' wealthy with psychic talents or a couple of births. Males who had a commonly glad upbringing, no data of multiple births, or no own family history of psychic capabilities or beliefs are least possibly to boom abilities.

Think lower back to at the same time as you had been a toddler. How modified into it? Did you enjoy quite some stressors developing up? Did a determine die while you have been younger? Did you ever have atypical moments at the same time as you sensed a few thing became approximately to appear or noticed things others couldn't? Maybe you have were given been raised in a own family that nurtured your gift. Now you're seeking out a way to nurture it, even extra, to beautify your existence and find out how you could live better with psychic talents. If any of these sounds familiar, you have decided on the right ebook.

## Chapter 3: Signs You May Already Have Psychic Abilities

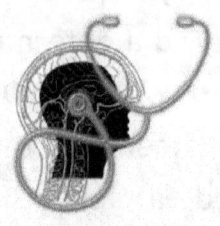

Have you ever had the feeling that you already have a few psychic talents or competencies? Perhaps you have got masses of research with déjàvu that you don't take into account are brilliant, otherwise you consider you studied that each time you as it must be are looking forward to a few factor, it's a trifling twist of fate. Are you responsible of ignoring uncommon sports that show up to you, or do you actually pause to appearance deeply? Many people who have already got psychic competencies in one manner or each different do not apprehend them for what they're, and so that they skip unused or worse, left out. Recognizing the capabilities that you could already have is crucial for this direction.

Why do People Ignore their Psychic Abilities?

•Afraid to be seen as"Weird": Our international does now not typically glorify or reward better seeing, which may additionally lead a few human beings to keep back their abilties out of worry of being seen as notable or weird. People do no longer commonly understand it when others see more than they do, and may resent someone who sees deeply into reality and is open approximately it. When you don't have pals round who recognize this hobby of yours, it may be difficult to pay interest for your intuition or live devoted for your route.

•Psychics are, at Times, visible as "Evil": At times, human beings with psychic competencies are even visible as witches, evil, or inquisitive about the black arts, which is not real in any respect. As said earlier, anybody has the ones capabilities, however most aren't aware about a manner to peer them for what they may be, haven't observed them, or in truth forget about them on reason. However, a few human beings may additionally moreover name the ones talents evil, if you need to guide some to cover their skills. It's essential to consider that those talents aren't evil in any respect and are only a herbal part of being a human.

It's additionally feasible that the character with psychic talents can be referred to as loopy or nonsensical if they may be open approximately their abilities or use them in front of others. It's a disgrace that we live in a worldwide that downplays such an vital and herbal present, however being aware about some of the stigma in the direction of the ones abilties will let you pass beyond being held returned thru it. Once you boom along your psychic direction, the ones judgments from others will not depend range to you as lots.

Signs that you have Psychic Skills:

For someone who certainly has the ones skills in a big quantity, they may only be held once more for so long earlier than they arrive out. Read over a number of the ones symptoms and symptoms that might mean you've got already got some of these capabilities. Perhaps you may understand that you're already halfway there, and first-rate want to understand what you have to be seeking out. Once you're aware about what those abilities appear like, you may glide onto growing them even similarly, or selecting that you need to awareness on. Do any of these descriptions fit you?

•Higher than Average Intuitive Abilities: Have you heard the cellphone ring and already knew who it become, in advance than seeing their name on the caller ID? Perhaps you can experience it while a textual content message is prepared to be despatched to you, or have stated an occasion have turn out to be coming earlier than everybody else. If you've got the functionality to enjoy whether or no longer or not someone has precise or terrible power from throughout the room, earlier than even speakme with them, you've got especially superior instinct. This is, as stated in advance, the first step on the adventure of uncovering all your psychic skills.

•Visions Occur Regularly to you: For a person with psychic abilties, visions can be quite ordinary and rise up regularly. If you've expected the future on a couple of activities, whether or not or no longer in goals or waking lifestyles, you really have a few level of psychic ability. These visions can also additionally depict what is taking place in the subsequent hour, or the following couple of months, and are huge at instances, and apparently trivial at others. In order to check this, start noting down your visions and mind of what is going to take location, to appearance if you can verify them in a while.

•Déjàvu is Normal to you: Déjàvu is some factor that everybody has skilled at least as soon as, however for a person with higher than average psychic talents, it's a commonplace prevalence. If you normally experience as despite the fact that you've visible this area before whilst you in reality haven't, or experience familiarity in new matters, locations, or humans, you are likely going through déjàvu. This is an indication that your psychic talents are already in track. Once your psychic skills are heightened even more, this might turn out to be an normal incidence for you.

•Accurate Gut Feelings on a Regular Basis: For a person with psychic talents, statistics what is going to reveal up in advance than it does, is natural. You can be in a function to inform how activities will play out, although it's quality a popular experience of "right" or "terrible". You can also be able to enjoy even as you'll get alongside properly or badly with someone definitely from looking at them, or in intense times, experience even as a natural catastrophe is prepared to hit across the world.

•Occurrences of Telepathy: Have you ever felt as despite the reality that your thoughts can deliver messages to unique humans? Have you picked up the mind or feelings of others seemingly without any strive? Perhaps you have got positioned which you are having a reference to someone else without even pronouncing one word, or have engaged in a complete communique with someone without speaking in any respect. These are all symptoms and signs and signs and symptoms of being psychic, and competencies that can be strengthened with strive and workout.

•Vivid Dreaming: When a person has psychic skills, they regularly additionally will be predisposed to experience vibrant dreams, which they will bear in mind even after waking up, in element. They see symbols within the ones bright goals that can show deep metaphorical importance to the dreamer, and moreover display hidden messages that pertain to what is taking place in their life on the time. A lot of humans clearly have desires that recur and inform a tale this is hidden in the subconscious thoughts. Tapping into this capacity can lend precious insights to your very very own mind.

•Sensing History of Objects or People: Being able to sense the information of an object or individual after touching it or them is some different psychic skills that you can obviously very very own. One way wherein psychics are so effective is because of the reality they'll be capable of enjoy information approximately devices, places, or humans by using certainly focusing. They every so often are able to hug a person or maintain their hand and revel in or revel in portions of that person's past.

•Premonitions and Predictions: If you've ever recorded thoughts down because of the truth you knew they had been going to stand up later on, after which seen them display up, that is quite obviously proof of a latent psychic capability. You should have recognised they had been coming from a dream you had, or in reality a feel that seemed to come out of nowhere.

•You comprehend at the same time as Trouble is Coming: There is a sturdy feeling that takes place while someone senses their loved one in hazard. This can purpose you to panic for no obvious or immediate motive, and cause a massive effect on you. There might be no on the spot cause for this revel in, aside from the overwhelming enjoy that someone near you is in hassle. In a few cases, you may understand who it's miles particularly, on the identical time as for others, you may genuinely recognise it's someone close to you.

•You feel Events from Far Away: This capability is pretty superior and tells you that you are definitely psychic. Perhaps as soon as you've got been both at paintings or at home, and will experience a few detail taking region from some distance away, both in some different city or perhaps america. If you've felt reviews from at some point of the globe and knew what became taking place, proper because it befell, you probable have very advanced psychic talents. This could have been some issue from an intensive, clean imaginative and prescient, to a robust revel in of trouble going on somewhere precise.

•You have Healing Abilities: Some psychic humans are able to touch someone unwell or suffering and be conscious that they revel in better almost immediately. Someone with psychic offers has robust and normally amazing energy that can be used to heal every intellectual or bodily wounds in distinct people. If this has came about to you, it's in all likelihood the purpose of your psychic competencies.

•You Predict Future Events: This one is quite obvious, but being capable of are looking ahead to destiny sports, telling them to a person close to you, then seeing the event truely arise, is one important way to tell which you have psychic abilities. These intuitions frequently come at the most sudden of times, and frequently without rhyme or cause, until the occasion takes place and makes it clear for you.

•Having Access to Sounds: Hearing sounds whilst no person else can, and continuously wondering why nobody is reacting to those diffused chimes or jewelry, can tell you which you have latent psychic abilties. These noises might be pointing to an occasion that is but to come back lower lower back. Some human beings with this capability are been capable of slim down what every sound method and use it to their gain, or to assist splendid humans.

Possessing psychic abilities need now not make you afraid or traumatic. These abilities are splendid provides and, even as superior surely, can be utilized in wonderful methods. Psychic human beings are very helpful and treasured to others that haven't started out to be aware or harness their private competencies in this vicinity. People generally tend to trust humans with psychic talents, even supposing they aren't positive why they bear in mind them. This can be for multiple motives, from guidance, to guide, to fixing mysteries, or perhaps a easy intuitive pull. When you learn how to consist of the ones abilities as advantages from nature, you could start to positioned them within the route of helping the arena.

A Psychic History

The first evidence of physics is going all the way decrease again to the Roman Empire. These humans had been called clairvoyants and may art work as advisors. Everyone idea that they had direct connections to the goddesses and gods.

The psychics may want to speak with the gods and provide the Royalty messages. Psychics were used to make essential picks. They were consulted about every selection. It didn't matter how minute or large. These picks might be approximately going to conflict, government moves, and planting and harvesting their plants. All of this got here with a fee. If royalty determined primarily based totally on the psychic's advice, and that choice grew to grow to be out badly, the psychic can be jailed or killed.

The feature of psychics grew with the development of civilization. When tribes original, Shaman had the psychic abilities. They had been the medical doctors for the village. The shaman had an critical position in their society. They have been at every ceremony to offer cosmic power. They completed divination, due to this they may look at the destiny for solutions, but the usage of out-of-body evaluations or clairvoyance.

Psychics commenced out the use of gadgets to help them conjure up spiritual strength. When their powers had advanced, they might use equipment like bones, jewels, crystals, and divining rods. These devices were used to inspire greater strength. Dice and dominoes are not unusual to be tools for advanced psychic readings.

Psychics superior the idea of actual fortune. They informed that there is not suitable or awful accurate fortune, it's far all electricity. This electricity is usually around you and can manage the very last consequences of high-quality situations. Most aren't privy to the power they launch into the area. This electricity gets pondered once more to them in both a nice or negative manner. This is why you need to discover ways to manage and apprehend your competencies.

When organized faith received recognition, they not commonplace psychic abilties. Christian, Jewish, and Islamic leaders deemed psychics have been evil beings, Satan worshippers, or witches. Religious leaders feared their capacity of foretelling and idea it would cause human beings to prevent coming to services. Foretelling is similar to psychic instinct and is the capability to experience that a few element is going to appear. The spiritual leaders concept they might be looked at as not having connections to better beings. This brought on psychics to be jailed, banished, or killed.

The maximum well-known historic story of psychics is the Salem Witch Trials. This came about among February 1692 and May 1693. A enterprise of young girls glad their whole village that a whole lot of their populace have been witches. It commenced out out truely enough with Betty Parris who have become 9 and Abigail Williams who've turn out to be 11. They started out out to experience "fits" wherein they claimed have been due to witchcraft. Both men and women had been killed for his or her so-known as work with Satan. One guy who changed into seventy one-years vintage changed into pressed to dying. Several died in prison of these fatalities had been babies. Nineteen humans have been hung. Many have been ladies. Around two hundred humans have been accused of being witches. The Salem Witch Trials had been led through The Christian Church because of the fact they perception psychic talents changed into insulting to their author. A new court docket emerge as created, and almost everyone had been given their sentenced absolved and their pinnacle call returned.

Psychics are a ordinary part of our society in recent times. That's now not announcing there aren't humans to be had who do now not take shipping of as genuine with in this form of hassle. Police departments have used psychics to help treatment cold times and abductions. Research has shown that psychics are actual and are an present day vicinity of have a observe. Studies have proven that psychic abilities are similar to the power in quantum physics. Psychics can be visible on many TV shows because the number one character. You can find out many books reachable on this problem.

Religious leaders no matter the truth that disprove psychic abilities. They continually warn their parishioners about the evils of psychics. They write them off as frauds, satan worshippers, or con artists. In spite of massive portions of evidence that those abilties do exist, psychics even though stay as unwanted visitors in maximum non secular institutions.

Intuition

Intuition is feeling like you're being pulled to do some component unique that can not be defined. Most human beings call this a intestine instinct. You would probably have met a person and right away recognize whether or not or now not you have been going to love them. This also can be notion of as an internal voice or better self that connects you to some element plenty large inside the galaxy. If you could calm your thoughts, this voice can come to be louder and clearer.

Psychic skills pass into extra exact records. It can help your instinct to assemble greater from what you experience to make subjects clearer and give you better notion. This records may be brought thru clairaudience, clairvoyance, clairsentience, clairgustance, or claircognizance. Instead of that intestine feeling approximately not liking someone, you will each realize some thing specific or see a few component particular about their past.

The first of the severa intuitive capabilities is clairaudience. This manner easy listening to. You get preserve of messages with out the use of your actual ears. Clairaudience is internal taking note of. You may possibly have had someone tell you some thing, but no character is spherical you, or the character you are reputation next to didn't say something. Psychics will pay interest spirits talk to them. It can be like you are reading to yourself. Sometimes, you will probably pay interest a voice in the accessory of the person who is talking thru them.

The 2d is clairvoyance. This method clean seeing. This is the maximum not unusual intuition. Clairvoyance is being able to see some thing at the side of your thoughts's eye. To simplify, it is like looking a movie in your head. This does no longer mean they are looking into the future or anything essential; it is also diffused. You can also additionally want to certainly see pretty a few, color, or photograph. You will need to decide out what it technique. It may in fact be a premonition.

The 1/three is clairsentience. This manner clear feeling. This method you get messages via feelings, emotions, and sensations. Empathy is the most commonplace form. People who're empaths normally revel in worn-out because of the truth they will be normally bombarded through the use of each awful and first-class feelings and feelings. You can also additionally stroll as tons as someone you simply slightly understand and may "experience" precisely what they're feeling. It gives you an capability to understand if a person is mendacity. This can be very available. If your skills are extremely robust, you may start to experience unwell even as you are round some of humans with awful electricity.

The fourth is clairgustance. This manner clean tasting. With this, you could flavor a few aspect before ever putting it into your mouth. Mediums on occasion enjoy this in some unspecified time in the future of a reading. When psychics strive to talk with others, they could begin to expand a flavor of their mouths. If the individual they may be attempting to find to obtain desired chocolate, they the psychic might probable absolutely flavor chocolate.

The fifth is claircognizance. This is plain understanding. This capability allows you to understand a few element without seeing any facts or statistics. You also can just apprehend that you may't accept as true with your neighbor or that new person you just began out walking with. These feelings might be sturdy and just pop on your head at any time. You may additionally have had some similar thoughts earlier than. You might have been reputation and anticipating an elevator, but something virtually knowledgeable you to take the stairs. When you get to the ground you desired, you discover the elevator were given caught among flooring.

A lesser commonplace instinct is clairalience. This is apparent smelling. This gives you the capability to odor past your normal capability. If you've got ever been sitting, analyzing a ebook, fun on your preferred chair and had been given a sturdy smell of a cigar, pipe, perfume, or any smell you could accomplice with a deceased relative.

These are sincerely examples of numerous intuitions. You do not ought to have they

all. You may additionally best have one or ,
or you may revel in they all at one
difficulty to your existence. It all is based
upon on how someone dreams to speak
with you.

## Chapter 4: Predisposition of Psychic Abilities

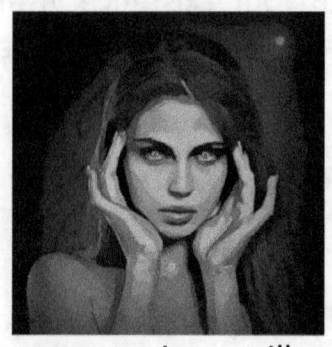

Psychic competencies will not play favorites. It isn't some thing that terrific human beings get. The electricity of a person's capacity has a big range. This manner that you could get a experience that someone is making an attempt to name you. You can also need to start to be able to take a look at unique's thoughts and feelings. Studies have proven that genuinely each person is born with the ability to increase their psychic skills. Ancestry and childhood moreover play big roles in whether or not or no longer or not the capability develops thru itself or if someone need to growth it on their very non-public.

Ancestry

A man or woman's circle of relatives information can play a huge function in whether or no longer or now not a little one is liable to grow to be a psychic. During the time of Shamans, a Shaman's toddler may get skilled to take over after their father's loss of existence. For some different instance of family playing roles in psychic talents, sisters Maggie and Kate Fox primarily based Spiritualism collectively. They have been every very advanced psychics. Spiritualism is being capable of speak with useless people's spirits.

Shari Cohn led a check in Scotland to examine styles internal families within the Highlands and Western Isles of Scotland. She observed that many households had a

2nd sight capability. They have been able to see activities in places in which they had been no longer at. Some had retro-cognition or the capability to peer the past. Some confirmed signs and symptoms and symptoms and signs of precognition wherein they'll see into the destiny. She located that out of the 208 people who've been studied, a large part of them did personal a psychic capability. She confirmed that girls are more psychic than men. If a person had a twin, or twins ran in the own family, they have been extra at risk of be psychic.

Cohn's research additionally confirmed that households who had psychic capabilities and believed of their competencies and recommended their use had lengthy traces of psychics within the own family. Sylvia Wright has confirmed this relation. In families in which psychic talents are not supported or believed in, kids will repress any talents they own. Children whose own family encourages and lets in them display very sturdy psychic skills.

A sociologist interviewed a psychic who informed her approximately an event she has as a toddler. She woke her mother and recommended her someone have become reputation within the nook of her room. Her mom spoke back with, "Did you ask him what his call is?" She didn't discourage her but advocated her to find out her capabilities.

Another psychic recalled how her grandmother helped her beef up her own abilities. Her grandmother might cover an object somewhere in her residence and informed her to "be this item, and see in that you are."

Childhood Trauma

Trauma that is professional ultimately of childhood helps to extend psychic capability. A researcher interviewed masses of psychics and medium over severa years placed that everyone they interviewed has a few form of personal trauma at a greater youthful age. The University of Chicago located comparable consequences once they did their interviews of psychics. This test confirmed youngsters who had tension in the family unit, had problem relationships with their father evolved a psychic capability. They had a terrific rating for the satisfaction they felt in life. This showed that psychic talents did have a courting with problem upbringings however didn't have an effect on their happiness in adulthood.

Science calls it the "use it or lose it" syndrome. We are born with hundreds and masses of brain cells. While growing up, if we do not use the ones cells, they die off. The research you've got throughout childhood can dictate what mind cells you hold into maturity. This will rise up in advance than they turn ten years vintage. How the thoughts organizes its cells is managed with the aid of way of how the cells developed. If children show psychic abilities, encouraging them will permit the mind to apply those cells. This will assist their capability to increase. If they aren't used, they will die.

When genes are expressed, proteins are produced those becomes genes, cells, and neurons. When a psychic infant is supported and helped to improve their abilities, this can make new pathways within the thoughts and lets in for extra development. Genes that assist psychic abilties are positioned inside the prefrontal cortex. This will increase in children who are clever and supported until the age of 12.

Psychologists have studied why trauma motives psychic talents. When children are pressured right right right into a demanding state of affairs, the brain will disassociate itself from the environment. It diverts the kid out of the conscious fact to shield them. Disassociation allows the mind to expose to exceptional realities and in all likelihood extraordinary worlds, times, and places. Adults who had annoying youth activities recalled having out of frame opinions as children. One psychic recalled that she suffered from physical abuse each day. During those times, she couldn't pay hobby or feel something. She knew and noticed what have become happening, however she have become numb to interrupt out the torture.

Another take a look at defined that youth strain triggered psychic capabilities talked with kids whose dad and mom were drug addicts or alcoholics. AL-ANON is a collection for person kids of addicts. This company often talks approximately special's emotions, usually their dad and mom. One participant said often he might probable come home not know-how if his mother might be handed out inside the residence or now not. He said that he modified into capable to inform what his mother's mood was earlier than he ever located her. He had unconsciously knowledgeable himself to have a look at her moods and mind so he have to recognize while she might be volatile or irrational. He had end up an empath. He changed into able to revel in the feelings and pain of others. Instead of disassociation, youngsters superior empathy as a way to self-keep.

Other predictors for psychic competencies are children who have been raised with the resource of strict, authoritarian, or abusive mother and father. Unloving parents who forced and demanded stylish obedience. If a toddler out of place their mom, has a extreme contamination or deformity that wanted many corrective surgical strategies, and children whose mother and father have been bi-polar. The possibilities of developing a psychic functionality are greater whilst there's a mixture of various stressors collectively with own family data.

Studies have confirmed that all and sundry born can own psychic competencies. They typically require triggers like stressor, early life trauma, or family information. This will take location earlier than they turn ten so the frontal lobe will thicken and lets in synapses and neurons to form. If the kid is sensible and possesses a better IQ, they may have till the age of 12 in advance than the frontal lobe adjustments. More girls psychics come from households wealthy in psychic skills or multiple births. Males who've a glad upbringing, no multiple births, no statistics of skills or belief aren't as likely to extend any psychic competencies.

Think approximately your adolescence. Was it an awesome one? Did you experience any stressors? Did you have were given a determine die at the identical time as you've got been very more younger? Did you've got moments at the same time as you sensed some element have become going to take region or see topics that others around you could not see? You might have been raised in a circle of relatives that helped you together along with your gift. Now you need to find a way to nurture it more to assist make your lifestyles higher. Learn how you could live higher collectively together with your skills. If this sounds like you, you have determined at the proper e-book.

## Chapter 5: What Is Psychic Power And How Do You Discover Your Intuitive Type?

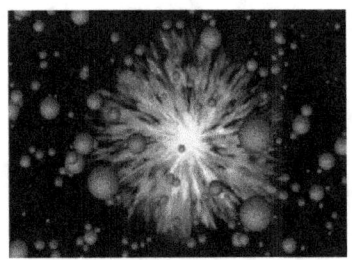

Real-life psychic talents aren't genuinely like what we grew up looking on TV. Psychics don't get a extremely good flash into the destiny out of nowhere, like a hint movie gambling of their mind's eye, simply in time to warn the problem of the vision so that you can change their destiny – the capacity to experience what the destiny holds isn't just the stuff of Hollywood. Although it's hundreds subtler than the manner it's portrayed on TV, it's extra of a heightened intuition.

Now, absolutely everyone has instinct, however a few humans's psychic instinct is stronger than others for some of unique reasons — the maximum common being that they don't exercising it an awful lot, as they generally don't bear in mind in intuition, and as a give up result, don't pay attention to it or can't discover it. It additionally can be due to emotional blockage or trauma that leaves you not able to tap into your psychic channel and focus your electricity nicely. Therefore, it in no way receives superior and lies unused and dormant in someone's unconscious.

See, your intuition is type of a muscle — you need to keep using it and training with it for it to alternate into actual psychic functionality. If you've grown up in an surroundings in which you had been encouraged to don't forget your "sixth feel" because it had been, you are more likely to have more potent psychic functionality. But there's applicable facts for individuals who were introduced up with the beneficial useful resource of the skeptics of the sector and/or in case you're a skeptic your self! Even if you didn't have this early publicity and permission to growth your gift, that doesn't disqualify you from undertaking psychic strength. For those of you in want of a piece of a spiritual workout, allow's get started!

One problem people who are possibly extra in touch with their instinct frequently find out themselves asking after they have a experience some thing is amiss is: am I certainly being worrying and paranoid, or is my sense of foreboding valid? The trick that commonly works for getting to the lowest of doubt about your revel in and whether or not it's simply tension or an actual premonition is: in case you sense a unexpected flash of foreboding or some experience that something's going to go incorrect and then

61

it disappears – that's your instinct. Heed the feeling and listen to what it's telling you, what it's caution you of. It can be gravely essential. However, it obtained't live prolonged, so strive your great to interpret it whilst it's there – you can even write down how it feels. If you get a experience that some element is wrong and in reality can't save you considering it all day to the thing where you're overthinking it and overanalyzing it to attempt to determine out what it way and the way you may treatment it to the issue that you're quite labored up and that it virtually gained't go away – it's much more likely truly anxiety and now not a actual psychic prediction in this case. It's smooth to inform even as it's anxiety due to the fact the feeling without a doubt received't leave you on my own.

Another signal that it's a psychic premonition will be a type of tingling feeling. Psychic premonitions also are typically found via a experience of tingling on your thoughts, commonly on top or among your eyes. They don't constantly come with this experience, however the possibilities are if something you observed you're sensing is observed with the useful resource of the usage of tingling for your head, then it's pretty strong to mention it's a premonition.

You can also experience very tired or low in electricity after a psychic premonition, regardless of the reality that this will be because of anxiety as well whilst you undergo in thoughts that stressing and agonizing over something can take a intellectual toll and make you experience exhausted in some unspecified time in the future of the day and later on. Hence, this isn't a effective way to inform if it's a premonition, however psychic premonitions do make one feel worn-out, particularly within the case of novices, as they don't realise but a manner to use the strength of the universe for help.

Using in fact your private reserve of strength is commonly now not the nice way to move approximately psychic exercise, as it's far constrained (instead of that of the universe this is limitless) and might/may be depleted right away. If you get a premonition out of nowhere (i.E., receiving a premonition irrespective of the fact that you weren't seeking to collect one), it won't depart you a preference to be aided with the resource of the universe's electricity – but if you are commencing to do a psychic analyzing, it is important not to use your very own constrained energy deliver and attempt the analyzing and to get preserve of premonitions unaided.

As you start awakening your psychic powers, you can begin to have a look at some changes to your lifestyles. This is a certain signal which you're at the right track and that your competencies are developing. Keep a watch constant out for some factor you note about your self that's out of the ordinary or if human beings say you seem unique. This might be because you're vibrating at higher strength now that you've started to awaken your intuition!

Vivid goals are one nice sign of this. You will probably phrase that the extra in tune you are with your self and your abilities, the extra remarkable your desires might be. If you're a person who no longer frequently desires the least bit, or not often recollects your dreams (and if you do it's without a doubt vague pictures and feelings), you may word an boom for your dreams, and you could endure in mind them more vividly. This is because as fast as your psychic powers have been woke up, your subconscious is greater freed up and much much less blocked, so dreams drift extra really. Being more in tune along side your instinct moreover heightens your energy, recognition, and connection to the spirit worldwide, that could present itself to you on your dreams now that your mind has been extra wakened.

Along with great desires and tingling sensations, you can moreover enjoy a higher frequency in headaches. If you do, please are seeking for advice from a health practitioner surely to be secure. It may be a sign of your highbrow capacities straining themselves and turning into worn-out from the psychic practicing you have been doing. The amount of energy you want to use to hook up with and hobby to your intuition and the psychic realm is first-rate, or maybe if you faucet into the electricity of the universe, it can although be a high-quality strain and a burden for a amateur psychic's thoughts to go through. However, worry now not – the headaches need to begin to dissipate as you progress and amplify your talents and come to be stronger and further focused. Eventually, as you emerge as greater experienced and in touch at the side of your instinct, psychic readings can end up like 2d nature – and at the same time as they're probable notwithstanding the fact that to be tiring, the headaches should subside except you are doing a in particular difficult analyzing or a reading requiring a first-rate quantity of electricity, popularity, and time. If they do no longer forestall, once more, please communicate for your clinical doctor about your signs. This is essential to hold in mind for all signs, aches, and pains that may be related to psychic studying, and so forth. It's commonly better to be stable and get them checked, as psychic ability is satisfactory one possible rationalization.

You may also moreover furthermore phrase that your special senses emerge as heightened now that you are at the path to psychic attention. If you've observed which you no longer need the subtitles have become on on the equal time as you're looking a movie, your pallet has modified barely, your eyes appear sharper than not unusual, or colours end up extra amazing, you're more touchy to sure material, and you can choose out up and pinpoint scents with a whole lot more ease, this will be attributed in your accelerated psychic capacity. After all, you're heightening your sixth experience; it's handiest natural that the others boom in functionality as well. Now, in case you get irritated because of the reality you still want your glasses despite the fact that your psychic skills are developing, genuinely bear in mind that becoming a psychic isn't a therapy to anything. It's no longer going to all at once will will let you see with 20/20 vision or give you a elegant pallet; it is able to definitely increase your senses barely, that's all. It's only a sign of improved electricity.

The greater your psychic powers start to show themselves, the better your vibration will become. The better your vibration and power become, the less time you will need to spend spherical horrible humans or doing awful subjects. Don't be surprised if, while on your psychic journey, your eyes are opened to the negativity and terrible conduct of some of the humans in your existence. This is a very regular part of the psychic journey, and you could emerge as feeling the need to get rid of certain human beings out of your life or cease doing fantastic horrific sports activities which you used to partake in. Unnecessary drama, rudeness, gossip, unstable conduct, and plenty of others., are all examples of factors which you may begin to have the sturdy urge to avoid or surrender. This isn't to mention you may't take pride to your preferred reality TV show now and again, or lessen a friend from your existence due to the reality they will be struggling with an dependancy or because of the reality they're having a tough day and get irritated at you or are bad in the experience that they're sad and perhaps conflict with depression. However, folks who are continuously constantly poor and want to tug others down with them aren't any person you want to be spherical. If it feels right for you and like it'll in the long run bring you happiness and empower you to your adventure, then it's exquisite which you eliminate the ones human beings (as lightly as feasible, without being impolite or imply about it, be polite and touchy if you do not forget they may be owed that) or save you doing those gadgets which bring negativity into your existence.

Negativity is tremendously draining to non-psychics so you can take delivery of as real with what it does to a person who's probable going to be quite at risk of the emotions, mind, and electricity of others. This is why it's miles amazing for psychics to avoid negativity.

An boom or development of psychometry is likewise not unusual for logo spanking new psychics. Psychometry is whilst you may enjoy the energy or statistics related to an item simply with the aid of using touching it. Eventually, you may without a doubt have premonitions associated with the object, but at the identical time as you're although a amateur, you could just be aware that you may experience the power of a certain item, often no longer on reason. This is quite not unusual in antique stores. Brushing in competition to an antique silver replicate, locket, object of jewellery, or any form of antique heirloom may additionally additionally moreover deliver you an unusual experience of longing apparently for no motive, however this will be due to the facts of the object or the item's owner. Perhaps the item emerge as given to them thru the usage of the love of their lifestyles who then died or left them or who probable they were forbidden to appearance. This ought to provide an reason at the back of the sensation of longing associated with the item. It generally happens with older devices or items that have been through masses, and whose cutting-edge-day or previous proprietors have been thru loads. It can be articles of garb, jewelry, artwork, furniture – no matter the truth that coming into a residence many psychics can revel in the power related to it and its information/antique owners. If you're transferring out fast and go to look at an open residence, to get a experience of whether or not or not the house is proper for you, moreover recall the power of the place. Run your fingers over the partitions, counters, and furniture in every room. This must provide you with an amazing indication of whether or not or not there may be a further of awful strength or now not, or whether or not or not you/whomever you're transferring with and the house may be an extremely good energetic healthy. You'll frequently pay attention of human beings's hair repute on prevent and having a enjoy of evil or terrible energy on the same time as entering a house, and then later locating out a homicide or some unique horrible event occurred there subsequently. This is due to the fact they are deciding on up the electricity of the space thru psychometry. People with extra advanced intuition and psychic competencies are more at risk of choosing up electricity, so in case you begin sensing such things as this at the same time as you touch them, it's a tremendous signal that you're on the proper song.

Four Types of Psychic Intuition

Now that we're discussing what your psychic instinct looks as if and some signs and symptoms that your powers are developing, let's take a look at the particular styles of psychic intuition and description them:

•Clairaudience

•Clairvoyance

•Clairsentience

•Clair hobby

You might not have heard the ones phrases in advance than, so here is a quick description of every.

Clairaudience

is even because it appears like someone is talking proper now on your mind. Not inside the same manner as human beings with high-quality mental illnesses – this is more of a brief way to a query, or recommendation, and it shouldn't sound/experience harsh or discordant. The phrase "clair" method easy, and "target audience" is from "audire" which means that that to pay interest, so you are psychically "paying attention to" the ones messages, even though usually, it is within the mind. It can sound just like when you act out a conversation on your head, or just like the way you hear human beings talking in desires. These sounds and messages can pop out of your spirit publications or from the spirit of someone for your existence who has died.

Clairvoyance

is whilst you notice photographs for your mind's eye that hold psychic significance.

"Voyance" because of this vision, so clear imaginative and prescient. The next time an photo springs into your mind, apparently immediately, strive to research it. It can also additionally have a symbolic (or very literal) which means about some element developing on your existence, or it is able to provide an reason behind a few aspect you've been wondering or traumatic approximately. Clairvoyance acquired't be a very unique flash into the destiny where you could see exactly an occasion an terrific way to occur as a film in your mind – like how they show it on TV indicates. It may be a diffused photograph or "vision" to your thoughts's eye. You may have had clairvoyant messages within the past without know-how it! Some examples of what is classified as a clairvoyant message can be hues, numbers or letters, terms, snap shots or pix of humans, gadgets, animals, locations, or a few thing symbolic.

Clairsentience

(easy feeling) is probably the most not unusual of the 4. It is at the same time as you experience a few element goes to take area. If you've ever heard a person use the word "I can honestly revel in it" or "this doesn't experience right" that is clairsentience. Clairsentience is regularly called your "gut feeling" or your intuition. Another problem of clairsentience is being able to experience the emotions of others. Maybe you experience a wave of disappointment in advance than your pal walks into a room, and then they let you know their mother has exceeded away. Maybe you're on the cellphone with your friend who has a broken proper leg, and you revel in a brief pain on your right leg, even earlier than knowing they broke it. Maybe you spot your pet and all of sudden burst into tears overwhelmed via unhappiness for no apparent motive, and internal a week, your puppy dies. These are examples of clairsentience.

## Claircognizance

(clean knowledge) is while your intuition helps you discern some factor out that your rational thoughts can't, a few thing you're perhaps stuck on. For instance, in case you're stuck in traffic, ought to you chance taking the approaching exit to get out of it and take the backroad, or will that emerge as taking longer? You inexplicably decide to wait it out and shortly internet web page website online site visitors has cleared, and also you're in your way. This is claircognizance. If you've ever heard someone say, "I simply understand" and that they have got no proof to expose their truth or no manner of information however grow to be being proper – that is claircognizance.

So how do you tell whether or not or no longer you're surely having an everyday belief or whether or no longer it's a psychic message? The messages and premonitions can regularly be quite subtle, but the manner to tell is if some element (photograph, sound, feeling, actuality) without a doubt pops into your thoughts with definitely no relation to what you have been simply considering. This might be a psychic message and not a notion. Usually, those psychic messages are quite robust as nicely, now not a piece afterthought in the back of your mind. However, from time to time they're quieter communications, so with a few thing that comes into your mind seemingly unprovoked, it's continually excellent to try to test it closer and analyze it – it is able to have a few psychic importance.

With those 4 channels of psychic conversation, if you simply take a deeper study the following sound, image, feeling or notion that springs into your mind unbidden, you could discover a few relevant psychic which means to it. The message(s) will help you advantage records, obtain communications from the spirit realm (spirit publications, exceeded on loved ones, and so forth.), or show premonitions or predictions to you, that your one of a kind 5 senses can't. You may additionally have already got look at this list and honed in on one of the four that you are feeling greater related with or that you count on certainly one of them will definitely come more manifestly than the others. Maybe you have used one or greater of these within the beyond, whether or not you observed out it at the time or not. Maybe you've already discovered which you have extra of an functionality for one than the others. That is likely the handiest you may be most powerful at and the channel you can gain the clearest nice messages in, at the least for now. I don't imply you can't exercise with the opportunity types and strengthening them. There are many psychics who, for example, commenced out off clearly gifted at clairvoyance and receiving clairvoyant messages, however as they practiced, they step by step have emerge as more effective at, and mastered, clairsentience and which have turn out to be their strongest intuitive channel. This is simply one example, but it's to show that you're in no way caught in handiest one state of affairs or skillset with truely one possibility! Although if you need to hold the handiest you have a knack for as your maximum powerful capability, then with the useful resource of all manner. Remember, psychic functionality is sort of a muscle!

Each psychic has a particular manner in which their electricity and intuition manifests itself, and it's frequently associated with who they're and what kind of person they'll be. Everyone, irrespective of capability, has one among four psychic personalities. You are either a spiritual intuitive, a physical intuitive, an emotional intuitive, or a highbrow intuitive. So how do you find out which sort you're and fits your psychic competencies? Well, every one manifests itself in a distinct manner, and there are positive inclinations associated with each kind that you could look over to aid you in discovering which one you resonate with the most, and which one appears to be extra you. There is not any dependable take a look at, however each psychic character is described within the following paragraphs – and with a piece of good fortune, you may get a experience of which one suits for you.

Physical intuitive are those that have deep attachments to important gadgets, and typically, psychometry (sensing matters through touching physical devices) comes evidently to them. They are people who're more likely to use objects like tarot gambling cards, crystal balls, palm studying or tasseography (tea leaf analyzing) to decide things about a person or the destiny and carry out psychic readings. They are very literally fingers-on with reference to sensing power, counting on physical presence or moving their fingers near an object or man or woman to get a experience of factors. This makes them those most probably to be drawn to the art work of psychic healing, or folks who generally have a natural information for the exercising. They are regularly homebodies and love organizing their domestic, fixtures, and decorations in keeping with their hobbies. Their home isn't certainly a few place for them to devour and nod off at night time time time – it is their temple and haven from the outdoor international, and it showcases a bit of who they may be. They spend a strong amount of time at home and frequently have masses of clutter and trinkets during the residence. They moreover thoroughly revel in spending time in nature and grounding themselves.

Mental intuitives are the analysts. They will count on subjects over again and again, turning it time and again of their minds till they find an purpose behind some thing until they yield a stop result. They usually ensure they undergo in thoughts every little detail, checking and double checking. They don't ever want to miss some thing, and they're now not big risk takers, nor are they very spontaneous. Mental Intuitives are much more likely to be clairvoyant or clairaudient and collect psychic messages through imagery or sound in their thoughts, as this is wherein they spend maximum in their time. They generally tend to "live in their head" so to speak and may bypass for hours on end with certainly the business enterprise of their personal mind, honestly wondering. They are going to want the most information and ask for the most element when they sit proper proper all the way down to do a analyzing for a person. They are those to right judgment their manner thru some thing – appropriate judgment, reason, and rationality are what they live through. When jogging on something, whether or no longer or no longer or no longer it is a psychic associated venture or otherwise, they normally have a tremendous capability to interest and live targeted on what they are doing. They also generally commonly generally tend to have pretty instructional pursuits, in spite of the fact that this isn't always the case.

# Chapter 6: The Art of Crystal Gazing Or Scrying

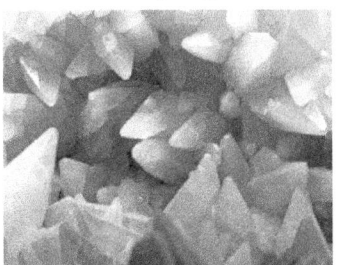

Crystal gazing, or scrying as it was once referred to as, is each specific herbal human potential that is straightforward to investigate as soon as you have lengthy beyond through the primary psychic schooling given in Psychic Development Level 1. Most human beings scry pretty really, never even knowing what they're doing.

Also, as hypnotists who use a focus for his or her artwork properly apprehend, as you stare right right into a crystal and input into an alpha or meditative kingdom, there can be a dishonest for masses humans to fall even deeper, moving into a trance country.

So, how do humans use scrying in their regular lives with out even figuring out it? Let me draw your hobby to many strategies you are using it your self already. Do you keep in mind lying for your all over again searching up on the clouds after which  seeing a female's face in virtually taken into consideration one in all them, or an animal in every other? That is a beginning shape of scrying. And keep in mind waking up in the morning, and at the equal time as your mind is lingering in that attention halfway among waking and snoozing and you don't quite recognize you're actually wide unsleeping however, you have a look at a face peering at you from the folds of the sheets? As you grow to be privy to what you're looking at you speedy try and popularity on it, and as your mind enters a everyday waking country and your attention adjustments, the face disappears. This is another instance of novice stage scrying, and anybody does it! It takes region simply whilst you are in that not-quite-huge conscious diploma, this is the identical of the alpha nation we require to do maximum of our psychic divination art work!

So, you understand already which you have the capability to scry. You definitely need to learn how to do it consciously, and to focus your mind in the route of seeing a selected detail in area of random devices and subjects.

I maintain in thoughts coaching a category on crystal observing decrease again in the 1980's wherein I forgot, myself, to focus on some thing unique. I observed an American army jeep visiting at some point of the barren location with a pyramid within the historical past and the Islamic moon and large call configuration overhead. I didn't assume a first rate deal of it at the time, considering the fact that I had requested no question and had no particular recognition... Until some years later, in Desert Storm and after, there had been many American army jeeps there. I changed into being tested a political future that I did no longer recognize due to the reality I had no hobby.

In scrying or crystal searching at it regularly is difficult to interpret what we see. To make this highly less complex, I constantly input my scrying meditation with a query, or a focal point in mind, which I write down. I furthermore date my page, thinking about the fact that like many distinctive types of divination, my scrying might also supply me a look into the destiny. In fact, it is the person of this form of divination to look at the future. Most of the stuff you see will relate to destiny activities once you discover ways to scry. Nostradamus is the maximum famous seer in statistics. He used an aventurine crystal ball, blended with astrology, to scry activities that might now not transpire for masses of years. But due to the reality his reputation changed into no longer precise, it's far not likely that he even understood his predictions himself at the time he wrote them down. Interpreting the ones pix that he copiously recorded stays the art work of untold numbers of students in recent times.

For me, writing my recognition down is vital to each keeping my vision heading within the proper route, and additionally to being capable of interpret the topics I see, so they'll be of use to me and the human beings round me now.

Sometimes the things you see on your crystal watching or scrying are real. The preceding photo of an American military jeep within the barren location is an example. This come to be an actual, real representation of some issue to move lower back within the future. But frequently the pics you phrase are greater like dream pix... They may be symbolic instead of actual. For instance, I can also see an photograph of a more youthful guy with stars floating spherical him. How need to I interpret that, besides I truely have posed a question? That photograph need to imply the younger guy can be a superstar, is shifting to Texas (the well-known person is the dominion symbol of Texas), is getting a marketing, or may be arrested by means of the use of severa sheriffs. If I actually have asked no doubt, I certainly can't interpret this photograph the least bit. I can in fact write it down, and anticipate a few element to transpire that fits. If I haven't asked a question, it's miles viable I won't even recognize the more youthful man. It can be a random state of affairs that takes place in a destiny now not my very very own. But if I actually have posed a question, I can interpret the picture relative to the query, using my revel in with dream interpretation as a guide.

This is one of the reasons I simply have advocated you to spend lots time on dream interpretation all through your psychic improvement research. Your dreams are a symbolic form of verbal exchange among you and your Higher Self and guides, and the higher you get at decoding them the higher you may be at interpreting the psychic records acquired to your readings!

Types of Scrying Tools

After my description of beginning-degree scrying mechanically happening whilst you shape clouds or do specific comparable sports activities activities, you may understand it once I will let you realize that you may scry in nearly something.

There turned into an vintage female on Long Island honestly everybody called the 'egg lady.' She used to take the white of an egg, positioned it into a easy bowl or cup with some water, deliver it a stir with a fork to create a few ripples and intensity, and scry out your destiny in one of the maximum accurate readings I've ever seen. She modified into amazing at interpreting what she noticed... But her use of the white of an egg in smooth water changed into a stroke of genius. Try it on the identical time as we have a look at the method for crystal looking at or scrying later inside the financial disaster. It without a doubt can be very powerful.

Water lends itself to scrying. As a rely wide variety of truth, water-scrying or water-divination might be one of the handiest techniques to grasp. This shape of divination is referred to as a Lunar shape (your scrying will sincerely be higher the closer it receives to a whole or new moon) and of direction the moon is related to water. I even have effectively scryed in a bowl of clear water, a bowl of water with a drop of oil and a drop of vinegar swirled into it, a bowl of water with a drop of ink and a drop of oil swirled in it, water with a drop of meals coloring and vinegar in it, inside the bubbles of a heat tub, in a tidal pool at the seashore, in a mud puddle, and in my morning coffee. I invite you to test with all of those whilst you studies the proper technique. Of route, you need to by no means overlook your safety both, besides the pictures you scry are certainly spontaneous, which does seem on occasion. When it does, as quickly as you grow to be conscious you've simply acquired an image, write it down and date it. If you continue to scry, do your protections earlier than you start to do it yet again.

So, manifestly you don't must be wealthy and be able to find the cash for a actual crystal ball so you can scry. Any vintage puddle will do! However, some of you reading this ARE interested in shopping for or growing a unique scrying device. Let me speak some of them right here with you.

Scrying mirror – These are easy element to make. Take any concave smooth glass dish and paint the outside floor flat black. You could make wormwood tea and rub the floor with the herb tea to enhance it as a scrying device. Wormwood is an herb that complements scrying. Or, you should buy a fancy scrying mirror and rub it with wormwood tea. The scrying reflect you are making will clearly be simpler to paintings with, because of the reality in making it you introduced your personal vibration to it. Glass itself is an insulator, so you will discover through and huge that glass balls, bowls or mirrors are difficult to paintings with initially, till you increase enough of an strength place round them, via use, that you could with out problem scry in them. An professional practitioner can with out problem scry in pretty much any floor, however a newbie does first-class with each a device he or she has made, or some element manufactured from natural substances, like crystal.

Real reflect – This is not my desired tool as it calls for that you learn how to recognition beyond your non-public face, which many human beings find out difficult to do. However, as quickly because the technique is mastered it isn't a awful tool. Remember, even though that a mirror is glass.

Acrylic crystal ball – I want to offer you with a caution closer to this. My non-public earliest crystal ball changed into an acrylic ball that I belief end up excellent because it end up regular with a flat bottom, and it changed into large. The first time I tried to apply it I sat staring into it for 3 hours (now not recommended) and got here away with nothing greater than a headache. It took many, many hours and years of use via way of my university students in instructions earlier than that ball evolved a robust enough strength area that it is able to lend help to the scryer.

Crystal balls – These are the maximum exciting. Crystal balls are made from rock crystal. These may be easy quartz, rose quartz, amethyst, or smoky quartz, all of which might be normally apparent, or of black onyx, aventurine, hematite, or unique opaque stone – most human beings find the plain stones less tough to work with, mainly ones with masses of faults and occlusions that capture the attention's myth. The very highly-priced perfectly clean quartz sphere established in all of the films is simply not as precise a scrying device because the much less perfect sphere or egg or maybe slab of crystal this is complete of cracks, bubbles, ridges, and distinctive imperfections that capture your eye and are with out problem transfigured into scenes and movement as you behavior your scrying session. The actual splendor of operating with crystals despite the fact that is that they create approximately their very very personal electricity to the session.

Crystal looking at, or scrying, takes huge portions of your power, specifically for the beginner... It allows to paintings with a tool that may supply some of the electricity. In time, as you discover ways to do which you won't want to artwork so tough at it, and it will take plenty an entire lot lots less strength to do. Until then despite the fact that, it's miles crucial to hold some time that you are watching restrained, and to artwork with a tool that both aids your strength degree, which encompass a crystal, or that at the least does now not take electricity itself to use (like an acrylic ball or a glass ball).

Selecting A Crystal or Scrying Tool

A scrying positioned into impact or crystal ball is a totally private divination device. It is NOT some factor that someone else need to choose out out for you. You ought to first test out the numerous sorts of gadget I've discussed, and notice which of them enchantment to you. Once you have got had been given narrowed it down, if the device you're inquisitive about are to be bought, you need to start to buy the correct one you want. Not all such system are created identical, despite the fact that they look the equal! The scrying device you in the long run select need to be some aspect that resonates to YOU... That you feel innately comfortable with. In essence, it need to be the most effective that jumps off the shelf and says, "I'm it!"

I don't forget clearly when I first positioned and acquired my personal crystal ball, a as an alternative small (about 2.Five inches with the useful resource of way of 1.5 inches) smoky quartz crystal 'egg.' (Yes, you are getting the concept... In phrases of crystals period does no longer depend range range, furnished the floor you're looking in is massive sufficient that allows you to see an image.)

I had walked proper right into a makeshift store that have been installation out of doors a seminar I become attending. From the entrance of the shop I appeared about 25 toes throughout the shop to a tumbler display case preserving crystals, and saw, from that distance, a miniature stagecoach whole with a team of four horses racing for the duration of the face of the crystal. I knew proper now it changed into imagined to be mine, and acquired it, not even thinking a as an opportunity hefty charge. I actually have by no means been sorry.

Most humans don't have pretty that obvious an advent to their crystal or scrying device. For maximum, it's far a feel of attraction, and while you hold it, (which you should do for a while to allow your own vibration merge with its) it feels proper.

Charging and Caring for a Crystal or Scrying Tool

Is there something particular I should do to charge or contend with my crystal or scrying tool? Yes, there's. First of all, as quickly as you have selected your private scrying put into effect it's going to grade by grade come to be an extension of yourself, as you operate it. You want to no longer allow special human beings contact it. Would you allow someone touch intimate elements of your self without permission? I perception now not. Someone touching or using your crystal or scrying tool is sincerely the same problem, as you may finally see.

Secondly, your scrying tool will in all likelihood need to be grounded and cleared while you first get it. Remember, many unique people, from its manufacture to its sale, have truly touched it, possibly even attempted it out. You will need to clear that vibration from it.

There are numerous approaches you can circulate approximately grounding or clearing it. (Incidentally, you would possibly furthermore test those for your pendulum if it want to ever enjoy dirty to you, or in case you need to have problem acquiring accurate statistics with it eventually.) The best way is to allow it rest beneath walking water for 10 or 15 minutes. In maximum times this is good sufficient to clean a brand new crystal. Or, you could soak it in water with three pinches of sea salt for that equal term, or if it feels very dirty, in a unmarried day. Or attempt burying it or letting it relaxation underneath a pine, oak, or ash tree in a unmarried day. These are particularly top wood for this, thinking about that each one useful useful resource the boom of the Third Eye outward as in scrying. All might also energize your scrying device as they ground it.

Crystal looking at or scrying is a lunar psychic capability. Your scrying implement likes the night time time, likes the dark, likes the moon. You must rate it with the useful useful resource of retaining it in your right hand as you meditate, at night time time time, on a entire moon. When you are completed, leave it on a windowsill within the mild of the whole moon to complete charging. Remove it from the windowsill earlier than daylight hours. It does not just like the mild of the solar. It will lose its lunar price if left in daytime and you may have to begin yet again!

Your scrying put into effect or crystal must not be uncovered to the light of day besides at the equal time as you are in truth using it. So, you need to wrap it in a mild darkish herbal fiber cloth like silk or cotton. Then, store it in a dark vicinity, like a drawer or a subject.

When you do your real crystal looking with it, you may find out which you get high-quality effects in dim lighting situations, along side in a room lit first-rate with the beneficial useful resource of a candle or a dim slight... You should have some moderate to look through, but constantly the mild will mirror inside the crystal and will become a distraction... You will need to discover ways to permit the mild this is pondered emerge as without a doubt one more imperfection within the ball or distinctive device which you are the usage of, and that you mixture into the picture you could see.

You may also additionally additionally rub ANY scrying tool with a tea of wormwood herb or yarrow to decorate its capacity to help you to scry. (Yes, this is accurate. The proper device may be a assist for your scrying, not a disadvantage!)

On Crystal Gazing or Scrying

Unfortunately, maximum of the books that I surely have look at on crystal looking or scrying through the years did greater to confuse my natural capacity to scry then they did to useful aid it. Most talk about the ball or scrying put into effect clouding over, and/or becoming hazy spherical the rims, and then in the end the clouds and haze disappear and also you see high-quality smooth snap shots, generally round the edges of the scrying device. This is puzzling at great, or maybe deceptive.

What clouds over isn't always the ball, it is your vision, as your thoughts shifts consciousness to the alpha wave diploma required for scrying. When you phrase a haze round the rims of your ball or scrying put in force, it isn't always in fact which you are seeing a haze, it is which you are the use of the gentle-attention gaze placed out in Psychic Development Level 2 to appearance auras, which uses the rods, in area of the cones of your eyes, and produces this hazy impact round the edges.

As a reminder, you bought the alpha degree by way of the use of manner of first meditating to although your thoughts, this is part of our protection and invocation of guides, and you operate the clean recognition vision by manner of the usage of searching obliquely, that is, in a roundabout way, on the crystal or scrying tool – this has the effect of first clouding the edges of the crystal, then making matters there seem to gain more readability. It forces you to look together with your eyes' rod cells, the black and white receptors, in preference to the cones, the colour receptors. Any colour you spot on your scrying tool (and you can see color) is precisely seen clairvoyantly. Your eyes will now not sincerely see it.

And while you first see photos appear out of all this, it's going to certainly be the imperfections of the ball or implement reorganizing themselves into an photo that your revolutionary creativeness is offering you with. This turns into a bounce off aspect to truely start to see photos and logos on your tool.

Now, study the subsequent workout to do your very first scrying!

Exercise #1: A Technique for Crystal Gazing or Scrying

1.    Darken the room and depart on only a unmarried dim mild deliver. Have paper and pen prepared. Have your crystal ball or scrying device set to go. Many people need to location their tool on a black fabric, finding this much less distracting than the tabletop they'll see via it. Sit easily at a table. Set an alarm clock for a 15-minute c program languageperiod.

2.    Be sure to reveal off the cellphone, and ensure animals and children are in which they can't come to be a distraction.

three.    Sit along side your backbone erect. Take three deep diaphragmatic breaths to ground and center. Close your eyes as you try this, and spot any anxiety or negativity in you swirl down your frame and out into the ground underneath you.

4.     Place your palms in your lap dealing with upward, and bring as a whole lot energy as you can into yourself thru them, and at the identical time thru your Crown Center and Third Eye Center. Breathe in as you try this, inhaling as lots power as viable. With each exhalation maintain to floor.

five.     When you revel in clean and all the manner all the way down to earth, located yourself within the white mild of protection.

6.     Put yourself to your protective strength balloon.

7.     Recite your prayer.

eight.     Ask for his or her help for your paintings these days. If you obtain an influence this is poor, you need to no longer maintain in recent times, or need to no longer ask the intended question.

9.     Now, open your eyes, and date your paper and write out your question.

10.You can also each pick out out the crystal or scrying put in force up or depart it at the desk and peer down into it or sideways at it. Experiment with function and location till you discover what is cushty.

eleven.Gaze into the crystal. Don't stare. Your eyes should be in easy-hobby. If you need to blink, bypass earlier. Allow your respiratory to become deep and regular, and to lighten up your eyes however further as you breathe.

12.If your eyes need to wander in the course of the crystal, permit them to.

thirteen.You may also additionally or won't recognize a haze over the floor and/or across the perimeters of the crystal. Ignore it.

14.If you understand an photograph off to the component of your gaze, do no longer bypass your eyes to have a look at it, truly permit yourself to join up the image collectively along with your peripheral vision. Continue to gaze with the same gentle-recognition hobby and make a intellectual observe of a few other pictures that appear.

15.During your consultation, maintain your mind to the exceptional of your functionality both on your question, or in a however and receptive nation. If you permit it to wander, the pics that seem in the crystal will both prevent or end up disjointed, reflecting your highbrow kingdom.

sixteen.When 15 minutes are up, deliver your interest lower lower back to the room you're in, exhaling deeply to floor your self all yet again as you do. Write down some thing you determined, precisely as you observed it, and in series. Be sure to put in writing down the reputedly inconsequential subjects, like a string of lighting fixtures, or your personal pondered picture which you might have visible. Once interpreted, even these things also can have importance!

17.Now earlier than you end, thank your publications for his or her help, and release your protective strength balloon.

Take the time now, to interpret what you discovered in moderate of the question you had asked.

Congratulations! You have certainly completed your first managed scrying session. In time you can become very adept at this, and it may even end up clearly one in every of your equipment of preference for acquiring future records.

You need to additionally phrase that exercising with scrying can be a beneficial useful useful resource to growing your clairvoyant capabilities to wherein you may begin to see human beings and logos round unique people, of their energy fields. And ultimately, if you decide to check spirit conversation (mediumship) it is going to help you to increase the capacity to appearance the spirits clairvoyantly as nicely.

## Chapter 7: Evaluating Psychic Experiences

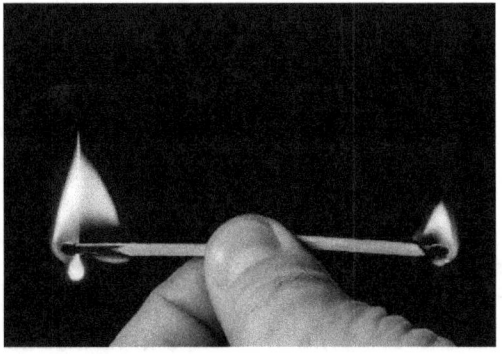

Do You Recall?

Can you undergo in mind your first psychic enjoy? Some of you could possibly don't forget it in reality, while others can also furthermore have very little popularity of any psychic experience in any respect. Chances are that it got here at a totally early age. You can be able to discover an older member of the family or acquaintance who can maintain in mind which you pointed out some incident which you have consciously forgotten. It could have been a series of situations or a single event.

All of those beyond reviews are stored to your unconscious mind. Even as you study these terms, you could call to thoughts a few issue that you haven't concept approximately in years. Some of you can have powerful memories associated with "unexplainable opinions" in your beyond. As you development thru those pages, the cause is for you that allows you to define and reconnect at the facet of your precise psychic presents.

Here are a few tips for in search of to take into account your early psychic memories:

Allow yourself to be open to recalling psychic reminiscence flashes, and don't overanalyze them.

Don't count on to get all the reminiscence right now.

Keep notes of your psychic memory flashes so you can refer over again to them.

Once you have an idea of a possible psychic flash, talk to others who might have been privy to it on the time it came about.

Use simple rest strategies to help you interest in your early psychic memory.

PRACTICE POINTER

Whenever you're connecting in your zero.33 eye, provide your self the inspiration that you may continually stop your connection via manner of starting your eyes, taking a deep breath, and connecting in your aware mind.

Count Down

As you rely your self down, you can sense your self sinking deeper and deeper, feeling an increasing number of comfortable with each count range. It is a completely first-class feeling, and also you sit up straight for the following range as you rely yourself downward. As you cognizance for your zero.33 eye, you can allow your self to loosen up more and more as you open up your psychic reminiscences. You may also allow any muscle mass that you feel are stiff to loosen up. If you are prepared, take a deep breath, exhale, and start counting:

5. Breathe outside and inside, and experience your self enjoyable increasingly with each breath. Let yourself lighten up your muscle mass. As you component out the following huge range to yourself, you can sense yourself connecting increasingly more strongly collectively together with your 0.33 eye. You may additionally additionally feel your self going deeper and deeper into your unconscious mind, setting out to your early psychic reminiscences.

4. Feel yourself going deeper and deeper as you revel in the connection to your

1/three eye turning into stronger and more potent. You may additionally additionally furthermore breathe inside and outside, slowly, exciting more and more with every breath. You can also moreover revel in yourself getting nearer and in the path of your recollections of your early psychic tales.

three. As you breathe slowly, you could revel in your self fun an increasing number of. You may additionally moreover sense your self going deeper and deeper into your unconscious mind. As you get nearer and closer to 0, you'll be increasingly more related together along with your subconscious mind. You can be ready to are to be had in contact together along with your early early life psychic memories.

2. You are becoming nearer and nearer, as you sink deeper and deeper. You are exciting increasingly, and your psychic

recollections may be organized so that it will get right of access to even as you get to zero. As you breathe internal and out slowly, you can permit your self to loosen up more and more. You can enjoy your connection for your 0.33 eye increasingly more.

1. You are almost there. You may additionally moreover additionally revel in very comfortable, relaxed, and consistent. You understand you may constantly come decrease back to a conscious united states of america of america any time you need thru commencing your eyes, taking a deep breath, exhaling, and feeling relaxed and incredible. You can also additionally permit your self to transport deeper and deeper as you depend slowly backward from 5 to 0, each quantity ten times stronger than the last.

zero. You can also enjoy the relationship on your 0.33 eye even more strongly than before as you are now ready to get proper of entry to the unconscious memories of your early children memories. Anything you see, revel in, listen, flavor, or scent will will assist you to do not forget your early children psychic research.

PRACTICE POINTER

While you're in a comfortable and cushty u . S ., you may permit your subconscious memory remember pictures from the past which may be about your early psychic evaluations at a tempo that is right and cushty for you. Be aware that you could open your eyes and are to be had returned to finish attention any time you want, feeling comfortable, calm, and refreshed.

Count Back Up

When you're prepared, you could recollect slowly lower decrease lower back up for your conscious mind. When you advantage 5, you will endure in mind any snap shots you can have recalled regarding early psychic opinions.

1. You are coming up and slowly releasing your connection to the 1/3 eye as you rely inside the direction of 5.

2. Breathe slowly and effectively, as you be counted range your self again up.

three. You have become nearer and in the direction of the floor of your aware thoughts.

4. Slowly launch your connection to the 1/three eye.

5. Now you could come absolutely again to the ground of your conscious mind as you release your connection to the 1/three eye. Take a deep breath, open your eyes, and exhale. You can also experience relaxed and satisfactory about your connection to any early childhood psychic reminiscences that you may have recalled.

Each time you carry out this workout, you may have great consequences. Don't assume a particular final effects. Each time you strive, you could discover extra and superb memories coming up to the ground of your conscious thoughts. Once you open the conversation channel and keep to hook up with it, the go together with the float will become less hard to get entry to.

Near-Death Experiences and Lessons

Have you ever had a close to-dying enjoy? Was there ever a near to call, inside the course of that you have been inches or moments some distance from capability lack of life? Did you live to inform the story a awful fall or a blow to the pinnacle? Did you have got got different disturbing recollections while you have got been younger in which your mind modified into an essential key to your survival?

Near-loss of existence research are to be had many one-of-a-type procedures, however going through such an enjoy can also have "leap-commenced out" your zero.33 eye into being more open to psychic intuition.

When you go through a annoying revel in, all your senses revel in a surge in the depth of the electricity in their perception. In a few times, your view of the arena modifications dramatically. You understand some thing's distinct, but you're not certain what it's far.

Children and Near-Death Experiences

A close to-dying revel in in early adolescence can also regularly pass not noted. Kids get into all varieties of hassle. They fall from wooden, get trapped underwater, trip down the steps, live on a vehicle coincidence, or tumble off the playground swings. In some times, this type of close to call also can moreover increase out of an subconscious need to break out a annoying situation together with abuse or an emotionally unstable own family.

A PSYCHIC TRUTH

Edgar Cayce had numerous early-life research that would have contributed to his psychic development. His skull changed into pierced with a nail at age three; he watched his grandfather die from a horseback accident; and at age fifteen he changed into hit in the backbone with a ball. This later enjoy appeared to assist connect him to his psychic recuperation information.

Can you receive as true with you studied of activities to your existence that might have affected your psychic potential? You are the sum simple of your lifestyles to this very 2d. Each new, passing second will result in exchange. As you discover ways to turn out to be in track together with your lifestyles, you'll be more privy to your psychic talents.

As a Child . . .

The desires you had to your kids want to thoroughly have been psychic in nature. Dreams, like one in every of a type psychic opinions, may also address past sports or destiny sports, or they will provide belief into situations which might be occurring at the time of the dream. Dreams are a wonderful manner to obtain psychic facts because the conscious analytical thoughts is at rest, and you are open to communication from your subconscious and your Universal Mind.

Think about the desires you had as a toddler. Do you keep in mind any? If so, are you capable of recall within the event that they had a topic? Did you have a positive dream that came about over and over? Can you become aware of the ancient term and/or vicinity of any goals?

Did you have symbolic desires that won't have made revel in at the same time as you had them, however which you would in all likelihood higher apprehend at this factor on your life? Did you've got any goals that recognized conditions in your life before you skilled them? Did you have got normal nightmares? Did you have got goals that have been one-of-a-type but followed a associated trouble?

Did you have desires in which useless associate and youngsters or others who had handed over communicated with you? Did you have got were given angels, courses, or distinctive beings or animals come to you on your sleep to consolation you and/or offer you advice? Did you ever have goals of flying or going to locations which you had in no way been before? Do you consider each other sorts of desires which can were of a psychic nature while you were a little one?

A PSYCHIC TRUTH

Here is an instance of a 2d-sight experience. Mary recalls that as a woman, she played in the woods with specific kids. They taught her a way to play their video games. It have become most effective later that she found out their games and clothing had been from the Revolutionary War length.

You can investigate the answers to those questions in a snug u.S., as you contact your zero.33 eye. Trust your intuitive mind to offer you the proper answers. If you can not keep in thoughts some thing, it's possible that you did not use desires as a part of your early psychic improvement.

Second Sight

When you've got were given been a infant, did you ever see subjects that have been invisible to others? Did you've got got "imaginary buddies" to play with? Could you find your manner to or round an area in which you had in no manner been in advance than?

What different evaluations that won't be explainable to others did you've got as a toddler? Did you ever have a go to from fairies or publications? Do you do not forget any contacts that is probably considered otherworldly, which includes with beings from another planet?

Déjà Vu and Learning from Past Lives

Did you ever, as a little one, visit a weird area and recognize you had been there in advance than? Did you enjoy a few element and revel in that it had already came about? Childhood déjà vu is a phenomenon that may take place surely.

As a toddler, your view of reality is first rate be- cause your early psychic stories aren't limited by way of the limits that society has set for adults.

Sometimes déjà vu is so robust that 2d sight engages, and the revel in will become so real that the individual having the revel in loses contact with fact. This takes region to a little one greater with out issues than to an person, however such critiques frequently stay with a little one into adulthood.

Past Lives

During teenagers, we may also nevertheless have reminiscences from our beyond lives; those recollections are regularly forgotten as we grow older. Do you endure in mind any early formative years reminiscences that might provide you with clues approximately your past lives? Did you recognize things about own family people from precise lifetimes? Did you ever act as even though your feature within the family were great than it want to had been? Did you ever inform your family tales about precise lifetimes?

Chances are, some of your psychic intuitions have come from what you've retained out of your past. The greater of those soul memories you can take into account, the greater you will find out a connection for your psychic gadgets.

Guidance from Within

Your internal steering system is your connection to the Universal Mind as well as the sum common of all the knowledge and research you've accrued updated in time. Remember that your inner understanding and research come from your soul and they transcend this one lifetime. The purpose of your inner steering tool is that will help you live on direction together with your life map.

Think of your guidance device as your ethical experience. It lets you comprehend even as some thing you can have said or performed or left undone is beside the factor. Of direction, you have got have been given the strength to override your inner steerage device, and chances are you do it all the time. Everyone does. Have you ever stuck your self pronouncing, "Why didn't I listen to myself?" It is awesome herbal to get stuck in the battle amongst your ego and your ethical enjoy. One is authoritative and looking for instantaneous delight, at the same time as the opportunity desires to do the right detail.

Building Trust and Confidence

It takes time to build take delivery of as true with and self perception in your inner steering gadget. It is much like growing every other ability. It takes staying energy and the willingness to chance making mistakes as you discern within the path of your goals. Many humans are beaten resultseasily and give up because of the fact the give up reason seems unobtainable.

The key to growing your agree with and self belief is to begin with one step at a time. If you simplest recognition on an impediment that is too big to climb, you can never have the possibility to get to the pinnacle. If you discern towards a small and with out difficulty feasible purpose, while you attain it, you will have performed your brief-variety intention. You will then have more self belief that you can make it in your subsequent motive. And in advance than you understand it, you have completed your long-term motive.

These small on hand desires are normally in music collectively along with your internal steering system. Each step of the manner offers a balance. Giving yourself permission to take a small hazard, and know-how which you have a safety net created via past fulfillment, you will become better and higher at achieving within the path of the unknown. There is a first rate thrill of adventure when you are travelling in sync on the aspect of your lifestyles map, in track along side your inner steering machine.

A PSYCHIC TRUTH

Your very very own answer can also come from internal yourself inside the form of a dream, or it is able to absolutely "pop out" of your subconscious thoughts. It need to come while you are imparting advice to others, and but the message can be for yourself. It ought to seem as a routine idea that you just can't get out of your thoughts till you cope with it.

Tune In and Develop Your Gift

To music in for your internal steerage device, you want to workout. The extra you reputation on growing your intuitive presents, the more they'll respond to you. If you can discover a everyday time as speedy as an afternoon even as you can focus on communicating on the aspect of your subconscious and your Universal Mind, you'll growth a addiction of connecting to your inner steering device. You will upload a posthypnotic thought that will help you with this automated manner.

If you would love to do this exercise, find out a comfortable place, every sitting or mendacity down, loosen your clothes, take a deep breath of air, and slowly exhale. You may additionally now reputation for your zero.33 eye. As you slowly breathe inside and out, you will be conscious that you have many muscle businesses; some of them are tight, and a number of them are cushty.

The extra you permit the tight muscle corporations to relax, the more comfortable you becomes. In a few moments you could be counted quantity quantity down from 5 to 0, feeling yourself going deeper and deeper with every wide range. As you pass deeper and deeper, you could experience your connection to your zero.33 eye becoming more potent and more potent.

Feel the Connection

As you revel in the connection getting stronger, you'll be conscious that you are receiving a beam of mild and energy that is flowing into your 0.33 eye from the Universe. This beam is good and effective, and it flows freely into your internal steering device, carrying the information of your soul.

If you're organized, you can start with the primary variety:

5. You are going deeper and deeper into the Universal Flow. Breathe slowly internal and out as you experience the connection thru your 0.33 eye getting more potent and stronger.

4. You are feeling the Universal Flow as it is obtained with the aid of your internal steerage tool. You revel in more and more snug with each matter quantity amount.

3. You might also moreover experience the vibrations of the Universe. As you go to the following range, you are increasingly more in song with the float.

2. You have come to be nearer and nearer. Your respiratory relaxes increasingly. You are going deeper and deeper.

1. You are nearly at the aspect of a deep and powerful connection to the Universal Mind. You stay up for the ultimate range as you're taking a few different breath and go deeper and deeper.

0. You are one together with your Universal Mind and your internal guidance machine.

Once the relationship is complete, take some moments to revel in the strength and peace of the Universe. You may think of many thoughts or interest on virtually one. If you need help or steerage or have a fear, ask the Universal Mind to offer help and confirmation which you are in music together with your life map.

Synchronize Internal and External Messages

In addition for your channel of internal communique, you've got an out of doors steerage device of old souls who've finished their life journeys and wait to help you. As Edgar Cayce said, the outside steering tool is an "invisible empire" that exists spherical you.

Your outside steering tool comes from the outdoor. It is a shape of outside communication from another individual or entity. For example, you may see auras or energies round others that permit you to achieve beneficial statistics. Or you could get a caution from a specific individual or perhaps from a geographic region.

Remember, those communications from the Universe can materialize at any time in nearly any form doable, from a cloud within the sky to an come upon with an animal. All you need to do is pay hobby.

Experiences of Synchronicity

One sort of outside steerage revel in is synchronicity. Have you ever positioned your self in the right location at the right time? For a few cause, exactly whilst you most want it, the cellular telephone jewelry with a method to a quandary. Perhaps it's an sudden amount of money that to procure sincerely in time to preserve off a economic catastrophe. It need to come within the mail, from a lottery charge tag, from an extended-forgotten debt a person owes you, or as a gift.

It can be very easy to overlook synchronicity. It takes place so really that it cannot even be found. It's like searching a magician cautiously so that you may additionally observe the trick. The magic takes place right under your nostril even as you are focused on some issue else.

You're Not Alone

Are forces like synchronicity and the alternative outside office work that your messages take all just twist of fate, fulfillment, or destiny? Or is there some issue else involved? Perhaps you understand that someone is looking out for you. Or perhaps you don't get hold of as actual with that there can be some thing in any respect.

Do you observed that there can be a being or a stress that the Universe facilities upon? Is there a divine reason or a better ideal for mankind to get in touch with? Is there a huge plan for the cosmos?

A PSYCHIC TRUTH

It's all proper to trust your very personal way. After all, that perception is already inner you. It is good sufficient so that you can examine whatever you study in this e book for your very private feelings. The critical problem is that it feels proper for you.

If you've got were given some thing or someone searching out for you, do you apprehend who or what it is? You can also recognize exactly, or you can have no idea. Just the possibility that there may be some factor creates the opportunity for hope. You can be cushty in a specific faith and feature conversations with the Divinity to whom you switch for steerage. You may match to the seaside or the mountains and communicate with nature.

Other human beings be given as genuine with in mum or dad angels who are stated to have a look at over us. You may also moreover join these angels to a person in your family or a pal who has exceeded on to the Other Side. They also can come to you on your goals, or you could revel in their presence, particularly in instances of need.

Whatever you believe in, the motive of this e book is to offer you an opportunity to discover your notion and boom your capability to connect to it.

# Chapter 8: A Short History Of Psychic &

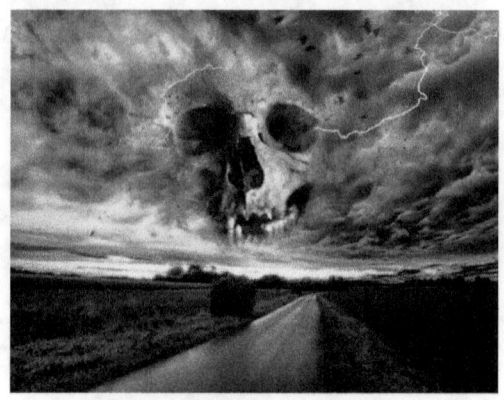

## Paranormal Abilities

Specific psychic and paranormal capabilities skip indoors and out of fashion from one generation to some other. For a good deal of records severa sorts of divination had been the number one psychic energy called upon or acknowledged through the not unusual character. It is only in contemporary instances with the preponderance of movies, books and tv suggests that different paranormal gadgets have obtained great recognition.

Today's leisure media are appropriate symptoms of the magical presents which is probably currently the most famous with the general public. Recent shows along side Charmed (1998-2006) had number one characters with powers of telekinesis, astral projection, divination, scrying, apportation, levitation, beyond vision, electricity recovery, teleportation and auric electricity energy. Multiple suggests over the past 15 years have highlighted psychometry wherein the psychic receives flashes of beyond sports through manner of touching an object that was concerned in the occasion.

Late 1800's to Early 1900's: Going yet again a few generations to the primary many years of the overdue 1800's and early 1900's, spiritualism and afterlife conversation have been very famous, as were spiritualist church buildings wherein contacting the spirits of the deceased via a medium modified into the vital a part of the provider.

Middle Ages:  In the Middle Ages there was a fascination with hearth. Even peasants paid hobby to the motion of the flame from an oil lamp or torch (lampadomancy) and searched for symptoms and portends of the future in the smoke growing from cooking fires and the crackle of pockets of pitch as logs burned (libanomancy).

Wizards of the early Middle Ages may need to regularly forged salt onto the ground and interpret the styles, or use a combination of severa styles of mineral salts cast into a fire and interpret the colors (halomancy). Casting pebbles or small rocks proper into a although pool or strolling circulate and noting the sample of the following ripples (hydromancy) have become some other famous technique of the professional diviners. A greater advanced shape of libanomancy, predicting the destiny based totally definitely upon the response of incense strong upon warmness coals, modified into furthermore a well-known shape of divination with the experts.

Talisman or Lucky Charms have likely been famous due to the fact the dawn of time, however have emerge as mainly popular inside the path of the early Middle Ages while it changed into now common to shop for an enchanted Talisman from touring wizards.

Another commonplace shape of divination at a few degree within the Middle Ages that has fallen out of favor in cutting-edge-day times is Mirror Gazing and related techniques using reflective surfaces, together known as catoptromancy. The psychic Nostradamus, from the 1500's, nonetheless heralded in recent times for predictions of maximum of the global's notable events he made that many people experience came actual, turned into said to want using a bowl of ink to exhibit a reflective ground from which he must divine his prophecies.

The paranormal electricity imbued in a reflect has been a primary subject matter in a couple of key modern-day and early modern-day memories, collectively with 'Snow White', in which the depraved witch sought a solution through asking, "Mirror, mirror on the wall, who's the fairest of all of them?" It grow to be also thru the paranormal capabilities of a 'Looking Glass', seemed these days as a replicate, that Alice journeyed to Wonderland in Lewis Caroll's fanciful tale.

Roman Period: From Julius Caesar to King Philip of Macedonia, statistics recollects the leaders and the records changing moves they took. But forgotten in the annuls of data are the psychics they consulted earlier than they took the moves. It modified into commonplace throughout every the Greek and Roman periods for kings, generals and landowners to are seeking for recommendation from esteemed psychics earlier than going to war, planting plants or searching out techniques to appease the gods for mistakes they might have made.

During the Roman Empire, observations of herbal phenomenon turn out to be famous, mainly augury, which studied the reactions of birds and home animals for the duration of thunder and lightning storms. Romans have been moreover huge celebrity gazers and often mixed the appearance of celestial meteorites with terrestrial thunder and lightning storms to divine the destiny (meteoromancy). Romans moreover had a ways less inhibitions approximately the human body than many cultures and often appeared each one of a kind naked within the common Roman baths. Perhaps the common viewing of bare our bodies delivered on the well-known shape of divination referred to as moleosphy, which made predictions primarily based definitely upon moles, birthmarks and pores and skin blemishes.

Greeks and the Oracle of Delphi: One of the most famous paranormal talents of all time were the cryptic prophecies issued by using the usage of the Oracle of Delphi in historical Greece. The place of the Oracle was considered a sacred shrine with the aid of manner of manner of Greeks. For most of its information, every u . S . Honored the independence of the Oracle grounds, making the shrine to be had to all Greeks and site visitors from unique lands. The shrine have become constructed round a fissure inside the floor from which issued spring water and an continuously burning flame of ethylene gas. It have become considered with the resource of many Greeks to be the sacred center of the area.

Archeologists say that the internet site of Delphi became inhabited beginning inside the 14th century B.C., at some point of the Mycenaean instances, by using using small settlements revolving throughout the worship of Mother Earth as a deity.

Over the centuries the shrine grew in significance and wealth. As it turned into fine open a few days every yr eventually of a 9-month period, and closed for three months every wintry climate, extended traces of pilgrims could probably form weeks in advance than the hole. Wealthy supplicants may additionally donate top notch treasures and works of art work for the privilege of decreasing to the top of the line and being graced with an oracle of the future.

The shrine espoused no precise faith and had allegiance to no particular u.S., even though it did have safety of severa kings now and again. Coupled with its geographically relevant vicinity in Greece, it became a meeting spot for intellectuals and a unbiased floor for adversaries to speak about treaties.

By the eighth century BC the Oracle of Delphi had become famous during the global places bordering the Mediterranean Sea and a protracted manner beyond due to the right oracles of the shrine priestesses, mainly one named Pythia. Leaders of just about every nation bordering the Mediterranean had absolute religion inside the accuracy of Pythia's visions of the destiny. For many leaders, any vital choices of impact end up handiest made after consultation with the Oracle of Delphi.

The famous Greek historian Plutarch, became born in a small town only 20 miles from Delphi and for a time served as a priest of the Oracle. It is from his account that we have an outline of the internal sanctum and the techniques. Plutarch facts that the priestess Pythia might enter a chamber in the inner sanctuary and sit down on a tripod that spanned a chasm within the earth from which issued small quantities of hydrocarbon gas (ethylene) which have been continuously burning in flame. Under the mind-changing have an effect on of the gas, Pythia might probable fall proper right into a trance and start speaking in a language incomprehensible to mere mortals. Priests which consist of Plutarch need to understand her phrases and interpret them for the supplicants.

The oracles have been famously tough to decipher, which allowed human beings to assign their preferred that means to the cryptic phrases, or assign the following sports to coincide with the prophecy, therefore insuring a totally high accuracy of the oracles. An example of the common dual which means that open to interpretation, will be "You will go you could go back now not in battle will you perish." Depending on wherein one provides a single comma the because of this that can be exactly contrary. "You will flow you'll move again, now not in conflict will you perish." Great information! You can visit conflict and the Oracle has prophesied that you could no longer perish however will move decrease back home. Or, "You will pass you'll go decrease back no longer, in battle will you perish." Bad facts; you may leave to battle however will no longer move lower back and could perish in conflict.

In 356 B.C. The temple grounds have been captured through an alliance of Phocians,

Athenians and Spartans. Its huge treasures collected from supplicants over many centuries, were carted off and purchased to finance their battle. King Philip of Macedon fast liberated the shrine and it fell beneath the protection of his effective empire.

In 191 B.C. The temple come to be taken over via the Romans and in 86 B.C. It grow to be once more pillaged for its treasures to finance a conflict. Three years later, now simplest a shell of its former glory, the temple become very well destroyed through a Thracian named Maedi who's the infamous man or woman that consistent with legend filled in the fissure and extinguished the sacred flame which have been burning uninterrupted for the reason that memory of guy.

Ancient Times: In the more primitive worldwide, any paranormal potential exhibited is likely to have been a exceptional event and led to the psychics turning into clergymen, priestesses, shamans and medicine guys.

Casting pebbles or bones and predicting the destiny based totally completely upon how they fall and set up, is a form of divination known as cleromancy that started out out in very historic days and persisted to be used in associated forms via each subsequent era.

Another historical shape of divining that might locate no beauty in the cutting-edge global is cephalomancy, which can entailed severing the pinnacle of a donkey or goat, then tossing it onto heat coals and making predictions based upon the way it burned and smelled.

Interpreting the death throes of residing human and animal sacrifices, and reading remnant frame additives, seemed to be famous types of divination in ancient instances as properly. Extispicy, Haruspication, Hieromancy and Hieroscopy, all which were prophetic strategies based totally definitely upon the have a take a look at of the entrails of sacrificed animals. As purchasing animals for sacrifice turn out to be past the way of commonplace human beings, they sought their symptoms of the destiny by means of manner of noting the severed heads and entrails of fish (Ichthyomancy).

The Old Testament / Torah relationship decrease again over 3,000 years, facts Joseph the usage of his psychic competencies to interpret the desires of the Egyptian Pharaoh. Dream interpretation continued to be a paranormal present relied upon by means of using kings and leaders via the Greek and Roman instances as well, and even though holds a few fascination with human beings these days.

## Chapter 9: The Intuition

The Third Eye

When it includes developing the instinct, the primary thing that might be discussed may be the 1/three eye. The zero.33 eye is

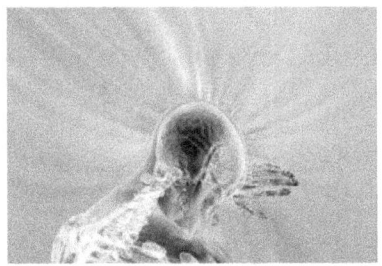

the seat of the intuition. It is the key to the electricity of clairvoyance, additionally referred to as easy seeing. The 0.33 eye or Ajna chakra is probably the maximum commonplace chakra that many people are acquainted with. It is what's going to assist you to see into the arena of spirits. Remember that the appropriate location of the zero.33 eye is proper among your eyebrows.

The suitable records is that everybody has a 3rd eye. It is simplest a matter of developing it, and that is a few aspect that you can do. Once you growth your 0.33 eye, you could have a powerful instinct, and you can moreover be able to access the Akashic records. It will depend on the way you rent it. Another exciting cause to growth the 1/3 eye is so you can see prana more in fact. There are many stuff that may be related to the 1/3 eye, but the most common of all is the instinct.

Every man or woman has a few level of intuition. For instance, have you ever expert definitely understanding who's calling your smartphone even with out searching at it? This is a conventional instance of the usage of the instinct. Of course, there are numerous other practical uses, which includes being capable of keep away from danger or really knowledge the proper course of action to take in a tough state of affairs. Indeed, growing the intuition can be very useful. Let us now appearance greater into enhancing this natural and psychic capability.

The 0.33 eye is likewise the pineal gland. It is a small endocrine device that regulates the wake-sleep pattern. In spirituality, while you talk approximately the pineal gland, you then absolutely moreover are looking for advice from the 1/3 eye.

Activate and Decalcify Your Pineal Gland

The pineal gland or your zero.33 eye holds first rate energy. However, just a few human beings can tap into this electricity and use it effectively. Many humans truely have an underdeveloped 1/3 eye. But the coolest news is that there are bodily activities that you could do to reinforce your zero.33 eye so that you can begin using and gambling its big energy. Let us communicate them one at a time:

•Who is it?

This is a few issue that you could do each time your phone rings or beeps. Simply ask your self, "Who is it?" Pay hobby to what you spot for your mind's eye. Do you word any photo or impressions? Be open to receiving messages. This is how you can connect with your instinct. You want to also understand which you have a robust instinct and which you most effective must analyze to connect with it. Of path, this approach isn't restricted to calls or texts in your phone. You also can regulate it a chunk and use it in incredible processes. For instance, if you pay attention a knock or any sound at night, you may ask, "What is it?" and be aware of any messages that you get out of your instinct. The important issue is to start connecting to your instinct all yet again.

•Forehead press

This method is becoming well-known these days. This, however, does now not work on each person but it's miles however really worth attempting. This will allow you a few specks of prana in the air. They typically appear as little dots or any form of white moderate. The steps are as follows:

Place your index finger within the location most of the eyebrows wherein the Ajna chakra is. Press it lightly and preserve strain for approximately 50 seconds. Slowly cast off your finger, blink your eyes round 5 times, and examine a smooth wall. Just consciousness lightly and try and see together along with your peripheral vision. Do you spot little dots or any specks of white light? This is prana in the air.

To help you word the strength, you may want to do this in a dimly lit room. Look at a wall with a impartial ancient beyond. This is a awesome manner to apply your 0.33 eye to look electricity, but it is not a advocated technique to reinforce the Ajna chakra. Still, that is some component that is worth attempting, particularly if you certainly want to look prana.

•Visual show

This is a high-quality approach to use for visualization physical sports. To locate the seen show, near your eyes and look barely upward. With eyes closed, have a observe the region of the Ajna chakra. This is your visible display display. You can project some problem that you want to this show show, mainly photos. You can bear in mind this as a few form of internal magic replicate.

The most important cause of this seen display screen is on your visualization bodily video games. Here is a smooth workout you could do to increase your hobby and power of mind:

Assume a meditative posture and lighten up. Now, examine your visible display display. Imagine an apple floating in front of you. Now, actually interest in this apple and do not entertain every other thoughts. This is similar to the breathing meditation. However, instead of focusing for your breath, recognition on the apple to your seen show show.

When you're organized to end this meditation, really visualized the apple slowly fade away and lightly open your eyes.

You are also welcome to apply every other item for this meditation. If you do not need to apply an apple, you may visualize an orange or possibly an elephant. The critical issue is to have a issue of visible recognition for this meditation.

•Charging with the fire detail

Remember that the instinct is related to the pineal gland, within the pineal gland is the 1/3 eye chakra. Now, this 0.33 eye chakra is related to the hearth detail. Therefore, you can empower your 1/3 eye chakra via charging it with the detail of fireside. This is a effective approach so make sure to apply it carefully. The steps are as follows:

Assume a meditative posture and relax. Close your eyes. Now, visualize the fantastic and powerful sun above you. This effective solar is entire of the element of hearth. As you inhale, see and enjoy which you are drawing the electricity from the solar. Let the electricity charge your 1/three eye chakra and empower it. Do this with every inhalation. The extra which you charge your 1/3 eye, the extra that it lighting up and grow to be more powerful. Have faith that with each inhalation, you emerge as increasingly more intuitive.

Keep in thoughts that that may be a effective approach. If you're certainly beginning out, it is endorsed that you quality do up to 10 inhalations within the starting. You can then upload one or more inhalations each week. You will recognise if you may execute this approach nicely due to the fact you could enjoy strain for your forehead in the area of your 0.33 eye chakra. Take be conscious which you have to now not simply visualize your 1/three eye chakra getting more potent, however you need to also be conscious that your intuition turns into more effective the more which you charge your zero.33 eye. The electricity of visualization have to be discovered through your cause.

Note

It must be cited that the Ajna chakra and crown chakra are carefully associated. If you want to decorate your instinct, it is first-rate proper which you additionally artwork to your crown chakra. Of course, this doesn't endorse which you must forget about your extraordinary chakras. Again, the complete chakra gadget is essential to your non secular development and to the awakening of the kundalini.

## Chapter 10: The Language Of Divination

Perhaps the maximum fascinating psychic

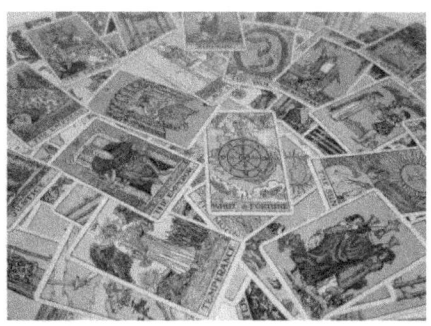

lifestyle is that of divination. Different styles of divination were in use from prehistoric times to the modern day, associated with everything from animal sacrifice to the analyzing of regular playing gambling cards. Needless to say, some of those office work are not every body's concept of an superb time. That is assuming you aren't the form of individual who might be willing to sacrifice a goat absolutely to recognize whether or not you ought to ask someone out on a date! However, maximum varieties of divination are an extended manner a great deal much less excessive, requiring nothing more than a deck of gambling playing cards, a canister of sticks, or a bag of tiles. These paperwork allow the not unusual psychic the possibility to faucet into their unconscious and advantage insights that would otherwise be beyond attain. In fact, divination can be seen because the waking form of dreaming within the recognize that it lets in the practitioner the possibility to get right of entry to deeper tiers of information just like a psychic dream. Additionally, a few of the 'languages' of diverse divination tools are very symbolic, reflecting the language of psychic goals.

There are some distance too many kinds of divination to cover in this kind of short area, so this financial disaster will interest on four of the precept workplace paintings used within the modern day. These forms cover fundamental variations of divination—single question divination and big image divination. Single question divination covers the workplace work that commonly produce a unmarried studying, which means that they may be supposed to deliver the feasible very last consequences of a specific direction of movement. These generally include such questions as "What can be the final effects if I take transport of this activity offer?" or "How will my date with so and so bypass tonight?" Big picture divination is a more complex shape of divination, given to exploring the dynamics of a situation. These forms frequently produce extraordinary readings associated with numerous playing cards, tiles or exceptional gadgets. Readers of huge picture divination will regularly get insights into energies on foot for them, energies working in opposition to them, and severa selections that the reader should make. These sorts of divination generally require a tremendous deal of have a observe a good way to draw close, and that they require the utmost of interest and devotion at the way to apply nicely.

The first type of divination to discover is that of single query divination. While there are numerous kinds of this exercising in all likelihood the 2 maximum famous and typically used are the I Ching and Chinese fortune sticks. Both of these types of divination come from Ancient China, and they function a testament to the mind-set of the Ancient Chinese. The common man or woman in Ancient China believed that the gods have been there to assist manual them in making the right choices at any given time. This intended that the spirit realm grow to be an extension of the physical realm, now not something to be feared or worshipped. Subsequently, the divine forces have been there for anybody, irrespective of fame. To do a reading in I

Ching or fortune sticks grow to be to really ask the gods for advice. The truth that the ones divination office paintings exist to at the existing time indicates that this outlook at the spirit realm can be very lots alive and nicely in present day times.

In the case of the I Ching there are sixty four hexagrams, or units of six-line readings. Each hexagram represented a story or legend from Ancient China, one which conveys a lesson or a message. To determine which hexagram changed into relevant the reader could strong 3 coins six distinct instances. These coins would possibly land heads up or tails up, and the reader would possibly use this to determine each of the six strains. After the sixth cast was entire the general hexagram might be located. The reader ought to then flip to the pleasant hexagram within the e-book for the message placed out. This exercising modified into applied in other Asian cultures in addition to China, and actually it's far stated that the Imperial Japanese Navy used the I Ching preceding to the attack on Pearl Harbor in 1941. The reality that such huge picks have been primarily based on psychic readings demonstrates how plenty religion the Eastern cultures place on divination and its capacity to provide course and data.

The 2nd shape of divination used for unmarried query conditions are Chinese fortune sticks. There are severa versions on this issue matter, but the most typically used format additionally offers sixty 4 specific readings. Unlike the I Ching, which calls for six precise castings of 3 coins, the fortune sticks require first-rate one casting. In this situation the reader has a canister with 64 separate sticks, every numbered because of this. The reader will shake the canister in a way an first rate manner to make the sticks slowly emerge.

This device may be completed until a single stick leaves the canister and lands at the desk or the floor, depending on in which the reading is being finished. Once the stick is identified the reader will flip to the best variety in the e book that includes the fortune stick readings. Like the I Ching, this ebook consists of unique reminiscences and fables from Ancient China, each with a very specific message and subsequent advice. Sometimes or three sticks will fall out right now, and on this situation the reader need to make a preference. Many people select to address all of the fallen sticks as big and examine all of the readings that they convey about. Others pick out out to area the sticks lower lower back in the canister and do it over again until high-quality one falls out. In the stop, there may be no real right or incorrect solution. The trick is to do what is right for you.

Single question divination is an great way to try and answer a urgent question in the 2nd. For the maximum detail those readings allow the reader to determine whether or not or now not or not or no longer they should pursue a sure course of motion. There are times, but, even as a better knowledge of a situation is wanted. For those events huge picture divination is a better supply for answers. Just as with single question divination, huge photograph divination has many paperwork. Again, there are some distance too many to cowl in the restricted region available here. Therefore we will examine of the most often used forms in lifestyles these days—Tarot and Runes. These styles of divination have origins that bypass decrease returned into statistics, irrespective of the truth that they aren't continually as vintage due to the fact the Chinese forms we've got tested.

In the case of Tarot gambling gambling cards, the earliest acknowledged Tarot deck is going again to the center of the 1400s. The motive of the particular Tarot gambling gambling playing cards turn out to be no longer for divination, as an alternative they have been real playing playing cards much like our modern gambling playing cards, containing unique fits and numerical values. However, as time advanced, the rich symbolism of these cards attracted mystics who had been looking for a medium for coming across know-how and deep belief. Eventually a system modified into devised which gave each card a selected symbolic charge, because of this that the Tarot deck became a manner to tap into the understanding of the unconscious. A extraordinary many spreads have become available, which means that any sort of situations is probably contemplated the use of the cards. There are 11 such spreads usually used nowadays, beginning from the single card spread which allows the reader to gain insight on a unmarried question, an awful lot as with fortune sticks or the I Ching, to spreads of as many as 8 or more playing cards. A unfold of 3 playing cards lets in the reader to advantage insight at the improvement of a scenario thru revealing the beyond, present and future. Other spreads provide deeper revelations, which includes energies that stand in choice of the situation, those who oppose the situation, or maybe commands that the reader wishes to research from the state of affairs to hand. The large Tarot deck includes seventy eight playing cards, meaning that there can be an endless supply of knowledge and perception to be had to the reader.

One of the extremely good topics about the Tarot deck is that it has lengthy gone via severa changes through the years. The earliest and maximum unique of the decks are though to be had in recent times, however unique decks with one-of-a-kind imagery also are available, because of this that the reader can choose a deck that first rate displays their persona. Additionally, considered certainly one of a type decks may be used to better represent the first-rate situation handy. While this could seem quite superficial in advance than the whole lot it definitely represents a completely essential detail of divination—the connection most of the reader and the supply of the information. Whether you accept as true with that divination is a manner to talk to the divine, or whether or not you trust it's far simply a way to tap into your very personal unconscious (there are people who should argue one's subconscious is divine), the crucial detail is that the medium represent your private imaginative and prescient of that which you are getting access to. Therefore, unique imagery alternatives allow someone to locate the imagery that amazing captures their imaginative and prescient of the supply that the records can be coming from. This personalization makes the experience all of the more meaningful, because it makes the reader a extra indispensable a part of the technique.

Finally, there may be the divination device known as Runes. Like Tarot gambling playing cards, Runes had been at the start now not designed for use as a divination device. Rather, Runes were the characters of the specific Germanic alphabet utilized by the Scandinavian and Germanic cultures in the technology generally referred to as the Dark Ages—one thousand-12 months time body beginning within the fifth century and completing within the 15th century. Different variations of Runes emerged during the first rate Germanic cultures, however the model this is used for divinatory capabilities is the simplest is privy to as Futhark Runes. Specifically known as the Elder Futhark, this institution consists of 24 specific Runes, every with a phonetic and symbolic price. The call Futhark itself comes from the phonetic charge of the number one six Runes, Fehu, Uruz, Thurisaz, Ansuz, Raidho and Kenaz. The first letters of every Rune integrate to shape the decision, really because the first letters of the Greek alphabet are used to shape the phrase alphabet—alpha and beta. While the Runes were at the start surely the alphabet of the Germanic or Teutonic peoples, they've end up a device of divination this is unsurpassed in symbolism and rich imagery.

Unlike Chinese divination, which uses poetry, legends and tales to hold understanding, Runes use greater primal images of their language. Uruz, for instance, represents the Auroch, a wild bison that included Northern Europe in prehistoric instances. This Rune symbolizes the raw electricity and strength of the Auroch, consequently whilst a reader attracts Uruz they are stimulated via the promise of strength that it portends. Thurisaz is the Rune for thorn, and it represents the limits that thorns can be. In the case in which a reader draws this Rune, they are advocated that the road beforehand may be whole of demanding situations, just like the rose bush is complete of thorns. Certain pains can be skilled within the path of attaining the reason. The simplicity and primal first-class of Rune symbolism makes it a fave for all and sundry who embraces a greater shamanic dating with the divine facet of lifestyles.

Runes can be take a look at the usage of the same 11 spreads as is used with Tarot readings. A single Rune can provide belief right right into a unmarried question, at the equal time as a 3 Rune analyzing can supply perception into the progression of a scenario. Other readings can recommend a fork in the road, in which selections need to be made, or they're succesful to indicate the forces working for and closer to the reader in a selected situation. In the surrender, notwithstanding the fact that there are best 24 Runes in desire to the 78 playing gambling cards of a Tarot deck, there can be however a really infinite form of readings that would come from a Rune session. The truth that there are fewer Runes makes this the oracle of desire for all and sundry who prefers a much less difficult, plenty lots much less complex divination tool. That said, the simplicity of the Runes must not be reason to underestimate their proper price. The truth of the problem is that Runes are probably the most symbolic of the divination office work mentioned on this bankruptcy. Rather than drawing on complicated imagery or written data, Runes appoint primary symbols to faucet into the unconscious mind. In a manner, Runes are definitely dream symbolism in waking life. To do a Rune strong is to basically have a psychic dream in conjunction with your eyes extensive open.